Pain Patients

TRAITS AND TREATMENT

Pain Patients

TRAITS AND TREATMENT

Richard A. Sternbach

Department of Psychiatry, School of Medicine
University of California, San Diego
and
Pain Unit
Veterans Administration Hospital
San Diego, California

ACADEMIC PRESS New York, San Francisco, London 1974

A Subsidiary of Harcourt Brace Jovanovich, Publishers

ACADEMIC PRESS, INC.
111 Fifth Avenue, New York, New York 10003

United Kingdom Edition published by
ACADEMIC PRESS, INC. (LONDON) LTD.
24/28 Oval Road, London NW1

Library of Congress Cataloging in Publication Data

Sternbach, Richard A
Pain patients: traits and treatment.

Bibliography: p;
1. Pain. 2. Pain–Psychological aspects.
3. Analgesics. I. Veterans Administration Hospital, San Diego, Calif. Pain Unit. II. Title.
[DNLM: 1. Pain. 2. Pain–Therapy. 3. Psychophysiologic disorders. WL700 S839pa]
RB127.S73 616.'047 74-5700
ISBN 0–12–667235–0

PRINTED IN THE UNITED STATES OF AMERICA

TO DIANA E. STERNBACH
WIFE, FRIEND, AND DARLING COMPANION

Contents

Preface

This book is intended as a practical manual for the understanding and treatment of the patient in pain. In a sense it is a sequel to my earlier work, "Pain: A Psychophysiological Analysis," Academic Press, 1968 (New York). In that book I reviewed the literature from several disciplines, showed several common themes which emerged, and derived some inferences for treatment. This work reviews the literature on pain patients (rather than on "pain") and describes our experiences in applying the derived treatment principles.

The case illustrations are actual reports and as such fail in being perfect "textbook" cases of the traits they illustrate. The case histories are of complex persons who reveal more than, say, hypochondriasis or depression. The original consultation reports have not been rewritten except for minor details to preserve anonymity and in some instances to provide follow-up information.

This book is dedicated to my wife, Diana, whose ideas and encouragement made it all fun.

Richard A. Sternbach

Acknowledgments

Some of the material included in this book was originally written for other sources, and I am pleased to acknowledge the following:

J. J. Bonica, Editor, and Lea & Febiger, publishers, "The Management of Pain" (rev. ed.), for permission to include portions of "Psychogenic Pain" (written with W. E. Fordyce), revised in the present chapter of the same title.

A Kiev, Editor, and Excerpta Medica Monograph, "Somatic Manifestations of Depressive Disorders" (to be published), for permission to use a revised version of "Pain and Depression" in the chapter of the same title.

J. J. Bonica, Editor, and Raven Press, Publishers, "Pain: Advances in Neurology," Vol. 4, for permission to use a revised version of Varieties of Pain Games in the chapter Pain Transactions; for permission to include a revision of Measuring the Severity of Clinical Pain in the chapter Diagnostic Procedures and Predictions; and for permission to include a revision of Conjoint Treatment of Chronic Pain in the chapter Treatment Methods and Evaluation.

R. H. Wilkins, Editor, and the Congress of Neurological Surgeons, publishers, "Clinical Neurosurgery," Vol. 21, 1974, for permission to include material from the chapter Psychological Aspects of Pain and the Selection of Patients in the present work, distributed among the chapters on diagnosis, treatment, and on special issues.

E. T. Gendlin, Editor, and the journal *Psychotherapy: Theory, Research and Practice,* **10** (4), for permission to use the paper Alternatives to the Pain Career in revised form in the chapter on treatment methods.

I am pleased to acknowledge the following for kind permission to reproduce their work:

Table I is abstracted from Tables 5–7 from M. R. Bond and I. B. Pearson, Psychological aspects of pain in women with advanced cancer of the cervix, *Journal of Psychosomatic Research,* 1969, **13,** 13–19; used with the permission of Microforms International Marketing Corporation, exclusive copyright lessee of Pergamon Press Journal back files.

Table II is similarly a summarization of Tables 8 and 11 from M. R. Bond, The relation of pain to the Eysenck Personality Inventory, Cornell Medical Index and Whiteley Index of Hypochondriasis, *British Journal of Psychiatry,* 1971, **119,** 671–678; used with permission of M. R. Bond and the *British Journal of Psychiatry.*

Table III is abstracted from six tables in W. L. Cassidy *et al.,* Clinical observations in manic-depressive disease, *Journal of the American Medical Association,* 1957, **164,** 1535–1546; used with permission of W. L. Cassidy and the *Journal of the American Medical Association.*

Figures 3, 7, and 23 are reproduced from R. A. Sternbach *et al.,* Traits of pain patients, *Psychosomatics,* 1973, **14,** 226–229; used with permission of *Psychosomatics.*

Figure 5 combines Figs. 3 and 4 from L. F. Pilling *et al.,* Psychologic characteristics of psychiatric patients having pain as a presenting symptom, *Canadian Medical Association Journal,* 1967, **97,** 387–394; used with permission of the *Canadian Medical Association Journal.*

Figure 6 is taken from P. Castelnuovo-Tedesco and B. M. Krout, Psychosomatic aspects of chronic pelvic pain, *International Journal of Psychiatry in Medicine,* 1970, **1** (2), 109–126; used with permission of *Internal Journal of Psychiatry in Medicine,* published by Baywood Publishing Co.

I am greatly indebted to my colleague Gretchen Timmermans, M.S., for the data analyses of our diagnostic and treatment programs which are illustrated in numerous figures throughout this book. I thank Janet Julian for her careful work on the illustrations. Elaine Cline, R.N., Marise Piper, R.N., Marguerita Moreno, R.N., and the neurosurgical nursing staff have provided enthusiastic and excellent service on the Pain Unit. Jerry Greenboot, M.D., was a thoughtful collaborator who helped form the Pain Unit as part of his V.A. Neurosurgical Section; and John Alksne, M.D., Professor and Head of the UCSD Division of Neurosurgery, has provided continued support. Turner Camp, M.D. (Hospital Director), William Coppage M.D. (Chief of Staff), and Margaret Harris, R.N. (Chief of Nursing of the V. A. Hospital, San Diego) have been most encouraging and supportive. Arnold Mandell, M.D. (Professor and Chairman of the UCSD Department of Psychiatry) and Lewis Judd, M.D. (Professor and Vice-Chairman of the Psychiatry Department and Chief of the

Psychiatry Service, V.A. Hospital) have also been supportive. I thank all of these persons for making our work possible.

I

Introduction

The purpose of this book is to improve the understanding and treatment of patients with chronic pain, by reviewing studies of pain patients, and organizing the findings in such a way as to be useful to those who deal with such patients.

The emphasis is on patients whose symptoms are understandable as due to an organic lesion which is not life threatening: chronic benign pain. Yet we inevitably also discuss patients with psychogenic pain, and the acute pain states. Much of the material is also directly relevant to patients with malignant pain.

There are several reasons for writing a book such as this. First, although there is a good deal written about pain patients in the psychological and psychiatric literature, this is scattered and not readily available. Second, the papers which are available generally make no attempt to apply the findings to the practical treatment of patients. With the recent interest in and proliferation of pain clinics, a practical application of the available information would seem to be indicated. Third, we hope that disseminating this information will help to decrease the number of patients who are harmed, rather than benefited, from methods of intervention which fail to assess properly the individual who is in pain.

Much of the confusion, and many of the treatment failures, seem to be due to mixing up the terms "pain" and "pain patient." They are not at all synonymous, yet many practitioners operate as if the patients are relatively constant, from one to another, and only the pain varies as a puzzle to be solved.

"PAIN" VERSUS "PAIN PATIENTS"

The word "pain" is an abstraction we use to refer to a great variety of different feelings which have little in common except for the quality of physical hurt, as in headaches, backaches, and stomachaches. Inasmuch as the unpleasant physical sensations vary so much in quality, intensity, location, and time course, it should be clear that only a special attribute is abstracted from all these conditions and termed "pain." In this sense the word is like "beauty," having no existence of its own, but having an element common to a variety of specific experiences, and ultimately defined only by the experiencer.

Not only do we refer to a class of subjective experiences by the word "pain," but the word is also used to describe the stimuli for the experience. For example, we tend to locate the source of the pain where we suspect actual or impending tissue damage, as in saying, "I have a bad tooth." By this we imply that the *tooth* hurts. Or children, when asked to define pain, may say, "Pain is hitting your thumb with a hammer." In other words, we tend to identify the pain experience with the injured or affected locus, i.e., the apparent source of the pain.

Finally, the word "pain" is frequently used, especially in research, to refer to a class of behaviors which operate to protect the organism from harm or to enlist aid in effecting relief. The behaviors may be verbal, as when a child complains to a parent or the parents to a doctor. The behavior may be a reflex withdrawal, as in pulling one's hand away from heat. Or it may be any of a number of physiological processes which accompany the presumed experience of pain and are used as objective measures of it, such as changes in cardiac rate or blood pressure, histamine production, or catecholamine levels. Such changes are considered to be operational definitions of pain for experimental purposes, or for purposes of objective clinical evaluation, and are referred to as pain responses.

Thus we see that the word "pain" may refer to many different stimuli, experiences, and responses (70, 71). As a consequence, it is difficult to come up with a definition of pain which is satisfactory for all purposes. However, Merskey has proposed a definition which is rather neat:

> *Pain is "an unpleasant experience which we primarily associate with tissue damage or describe in terms of tissue damage or both* (53, p. 21)."

In this one sentence, there is reference to the subjective experience, the apparent stimulus, and the objective response by which an observer would know that another was in pain. It is a definition which is particularly useful for our clinical purposes, because we will be considering in some detail what people say and do about their pain experiences.

We need to emphasize, however, the difference between "pain" and "pain patients." "Pain," as we have been describing it, is an abstract concept which refers to different specific unpleasant experiences associated with different kinds of tissue damage. Thousands of papers and monographs have been written about studies on pain, seeking to explain the mechanisms by which it occurs, and how to relieve it.

On the other hand, relatively little has been written about pain patients, who are real individual persons. As we will be using the term, "pain patients" refers to those who present themselves to doctors with a complaint of pain, seeking relief from it. In particular, we will be referring most often to those whose complaint is chronic, i.e., persists constantly or intermittently for several months or more. And as we already indicated, we will be emphasizing the problems of those whose pain is "benign," rather than those whose pain is associated with a life-threatening disease. This is because the former must learn again how to live, while the latter must learn how to die, and far more has been written about helping patients to face dying than about helping patients to face living with pain.

Compared with the voluminous literature on pain, what has been written about pain patients is rather meager. This is surprising and unfortunate, because doctors must, after all, treat pain patients. It is true that the doctor may think of his task as that of diagnosing and relieving *pain,* and in many instances he is able to do so quite well. However, the fact that there are millions of unfortunate persons who persist in seeking relief from pain, which is not forthcoming, suggests that the problem is not so simple, and that understanding pain may not be sufficient for treating pain patients.

The studies of pain patients, although relatively few and scattered, are now sufficient to provide us with an outline of recurrent themes and patterns. Pain patients are all different individuals, yet they share certain characteristics by virtue of being in chronic pain. When these characteristics are known, they will help the doctor to understand the individual patient and therefore to treat him more successfully.

Throughout the book, the word "doctor" is used nonspecifically. Most often it will be seen, in context, to refer to the medical person, physician, or surgeon, who is most likely to be faced with the pain patient, and least likely to be aware of the literature about him. At other times, it is clear that the word "doctor" refers to the general psychiatrist or clinical psychologist who may be called upon to consult in the evaluation of a patient, or to be responsible for the management of his care. Such doctors are generally more familiar with psychiatric patients, and need some references to help in making appropriate diagnoses and treatment recommendations when dealing with pain patients.

The plan of this book is as follows. We begin with a composite description of the subjective experience of the person in chronic pain. This provides us with some appreciation of what such a person lives through, and it also provides some clues about psychological traits—with implications for assessment and management—which foreshadow material in later sections. We then consider studies of the effects of chronic pain on psychological functioning, and then highlight the portrait which emerges by turning the inquiry around and examining patients whose pain is best explained in psychological terms. This done, we are then able to consider certain of the major features of pain patients, and then the implications for their evaluation and treatment.

There is some new information in the final chapters of this book because relatively few have committed themselves to the systematic treatment of pain patients with objective evaluation of results, and the few clinical investigators who have done so have not yet published all their findings at the time of this writing. Consequently, although we cite some of our own work which is published or in press, we are nevertheless forced to present some new material, for illustrative purposes, which is still preliminary and in need of confirmation. This is clearly stated at the appropriate places in the text.

Despite the relative lack of objective studies of diagnostic and treatment processes, it would seem that we know a good deal more about chronic pain patients than we have let ourselves realize, and we can do more for them than we have thus far.

II

The Experience of Chronic Pain

Most of us have had experience with pain, but it has usually been acute pain—short-lasting, or easily reversible. We may have experienced a toothache, or stomachache, or headache, or a sprain or muscle cramp. We took appropriate action ourselves, or sought out a doctor, and the pain went away.

In such instances the pain was a response to tissue damage, actual or impending, and served as a warning signal which caused us to take care of ourselves.

If the pain did not come on too quickly, there may have been some initial uncomfortable feelings, some twinges or sensations of fullness. These we may have just barely noticed and then pushed out of awareness as we went on about our activities.

Then as the sensations became more intense and crossed the threshold to become mild pain, we were forced to focus on the pain. With this awareness came a sudden alarm or mild anxiety, a concern for what might be wrong. Is something broken? Are we ill—do we have a fever? We feel impelled to impose a cognitive structure on this experience, to understand it. When we do so the initial anxiety dissipates. "It is only a sprain, nothing seems broken." Or, "It is only that tooth again, I'll probably have to make an appointment with the dentist." Or, "I'm getting a headache, the tension must be getting to me."

If, however, the pain persists and increases in intensity, we are taken by a new alarm and somewhat greater anxiety. It consists of two parts. There is a concern that our understanding for the pain may be mistaken, that it may represent something more serious than we suspected: "Say, something's really wrong!" And there is a fear that the pain is going to increase in severity and get beyond control. This latter can be particularly upsetting, for with increasing pain, there is a tendency to assume that the rate of increase of pain intensity is likely to be constant. (In experimental tests, it very nearly is, but our upper tolerance for pain is greater than we anticipate it to be, see Ref. 77.)

These reactions to the acute pain situation are illustrated in Fig. 1. It shows that as pain increases so does our anxiety, until, at a certain point, we do something to obtain relief before the pain becomes very severe.

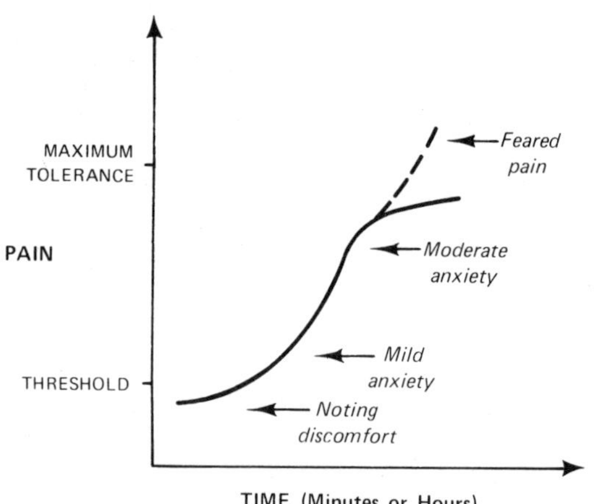

Fig. 1. Sequence of reactions to acute pain.

This is the experience most of us have had with acute pain, and we tend to generalize our experience to all pain conditions. However, the experience with chronic pain is quite different. The pain which persists causes the defensive reflexes to diminish because they do not help. Help-seeking behavior becomes more urgent, more desperate, and yet more routinized and hopeless.

As examples of chronic benign pain states we may think of low-back pain and sciatica, or other disc syndromes; causalgia, or other peripheral nerve neuropathies; arthritis; thalamic pain, trigeminal neuralgia, or other central pain states, etc. Patients with these diseases usually experience constant pain, which may wax and wane in intensity but seldom disappears completely.

One important difference between the acute and the chronic pain experience is that the patient cannot give meaning to the chronic pain. He may "understand" it in the sense that he has been given an explanation by his doctor, but the pain makes no sense as a warning signal, since it cannot be avoided or treated. Even when the underlying disease or pathology can be specified quite precisely (which is not always the case), there may be no effective treatment. It is in this sense that the pain is meaningless, as compared with the meaning that we can give to the acute pain which leads us to take appropriate pain-relieving action.

There is another sense in which the pain patient finds it difficult to ascribe meaning to his pain, and that is in trying to find a purpose for it. In acute pain states, we can blame our carelessness for a sprained ankle, for not visiting the dentist earlier, for eating something we shouldn't have, etc. But how can we "deserve" constant pain? Pain is associated in our minds with punishment for carelessness or wrongdoing when we were children, and as adults the experience of pain causes us to seek to find something we did to bring on the pain. "Why me?," the patient asks himself, as he tries to find some way of atoning or undoing so that he can get relief. And as there is seldom a reason "why," the patient experiences both a certain amount of confusion as to the meaning for his suffering, and a bitterness that others who are more wicked or sinful seem to be enjoying their lives without pain.

In addition to the meaninglessness of his pain, the chronic pain patient experiences despair at the seeming endlessness of his suffering. No time limit is set, and he sees his future as a hell in which he continues to have pain as intense as or worse than that which he now endures, with only death providing relief. The anxiety which accompanies acute pain is thus replaced by visions of a bleak, dismal future leading to feelings of hopelessness and despair.

Le Shan (41) has pointed out that these attributes of meaninglessness, helplessness, and hopelessness are characteristic of the nightmare, and the patient in chronic pain lives every day in the unreal world of the nightmare. A similar feeling was expressed to me by a patient who said, "It's always three o'clock in the morning."

Three o'clock in the morning is a very lonely time. Not only does the patient in chronic pain have difficulty getting to sleep, but his pain usually awakens him during the night. At this time others are usually sleeping, and there is little the patient can do to distract himself without awakening the others. Besides, if he did awaken them it would not help him much, as there is little or nothing that they could do to relieve his pain. So the patient is essentially forced to lie awake with little to do but think about his pain, and worry about it.

The worry takes the form of: "What if?" "What if the doctors have missed something, and the pain is due to something more serious like cancer?" "What if the pain gets worse? I can barely take it now." "What if I can't go back to work, how will I live?" Etc. These sorts of worries would, by themselves, be enough to keep the patient awake; combined with the pain, they make inadequate sleep virtually a certainty. The patient has few distractions at night and so the pain seems worse; he is forced to focus on it and that makes it seem worse still; he worries about it and so it seems still more intense, which worries him more. Thus, the night becomes a spiralling horrible experience, and every improbable fear becomes a dreaded possibility.

Pain patients frequently say that they could stand their pain much better if they could only get a good night's sleep. They feel as though their resistance is weakened by their lack of sleep. They never feel rested. They feel worn down, worn out, exhausted. They find themselves getting more and more irritable with their families, they have fewer and fewer friends, and fewer and fewer interests. Gradually, as time goes on, the boundaries of their world seem to shrink. They become more and more preoccupied with their pain, less and less interested in the world around them. Their world begins to center around home, doctor's office, and pharmacy. With this centering, the pain seems to become more unbearable.

The difference between this experience, and the experience of acute pain, is diagramed in Fig. 2. Here, it will be noticed, the time scale is not in minutes or hours, but in months and years. Furthermore, it seems to the patient, as he looks back over his illness, that his pain has gotten progressively worse, despite periodic improvements. Whether this is so from a physiological point of view, or merely seems that way to him, is neither answerable nor important.

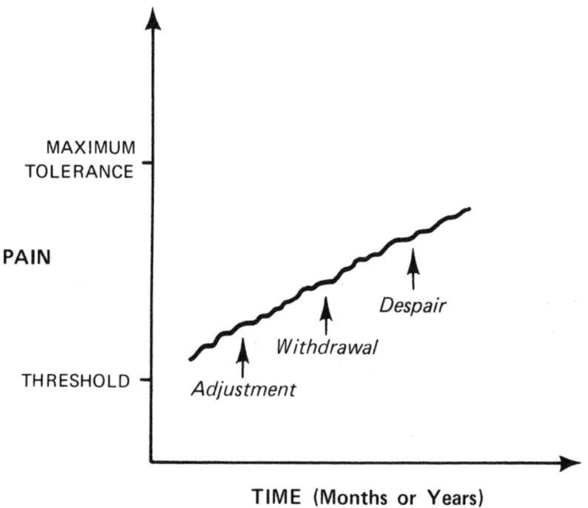

Fig. 2. Sequence of reactions to chronic pain.

Another feature of the chronic pain patient's experience is his dealings with doctors. Initially he will probably have consulted a family physician or general practitioner, who after a period of time will have referred the patient to a specialist. The patient will have been hospitalized several times for extensive diagnostic procedures. As his disease is diagnosed and the underlying pathology is found not to be treatable, the patient makes his way finally to the neurologist and neurosurgeon for consultations on methods of pain control.

The patient is in the position of requesting pain relief. The doctors are in the unfortunate position of not having much to offer, surprisingly enough. There are drastic measures which afford quite dramatic relief in the short run, say for the cancer patient who has a few months to live. But for the patient with severe benign pain, who has many years to live, there are few possibilities. Analgesics lose their effectiveness, and in the many instances in which neurosurgery is feasible, the pain gradually returns to its former intensity.

Consequently, the patient is frequently placed on the smallest possible dosages of a combination of medications, and instructed to return for follow-up visits at frequent and regular intervals. The medications seldom eliminate the pain, or reduce it significantly; at best they "just barely take the edge off it," and at each follow-up visit the patient finds himself requesting more pills for pain relief and for sleep. The number and potency of these pills increase until nothing works very well, the patient is desperate, and the doctor is alarmed at the addiction problem.

The patient is admitted again to a hospital to be detoxified—withdrawn to the smallest possible dosages of the weakest possible medications. At this time a new round of consultations is requested, and the consultants may include a psychiatrist or psychologist. The meeting is seldom auspicious, and would be comical if it were not so tragic.

The pain patient has now been suffering for several months or years, and has seen dozens of doctors who have all asked pretty much the same questions. The patient is now being withdrawn from narcotics, and in addition to hurting more than usual, he is feeling much more irritable and edgy than usual. When the psychologist or psychiatrist comes in and introduces himself, the patient is shocked and angry. He knows he is not crazy or imagining his pain, and he knows he is not a drug addict but needs the analgesics to control his pain. The patient feels betrayed by his doctor who has sent for this "head-shrinker."

The "head-shrinker," for his part, will do his best to soothe the patient's feelings, and will try to determine whether the patient is crazy or a drug addict, or if the pain is "psychosomatic," that is, a symptom of an emotional stress as are many cases of, for example, headaches or ulcers. These will all prove not to be the case, and this consultant will leave with few helpful recommendations. The patient will be left with some concern that his case must be more hopeless than he feared, especially if his doctor felt it necessary to send for the psychiatrist.

Finally the patient is sent home with a new set of prescriptions and an appointment for an office visit, and the sequence begins anew. The patient thus acquires a new set of feelings and attitudes. He experiences frequent hopefulness and then disappointment, and gradually feels increasing bitterness and resentment towards the doctors who examine him, poking and sticking and asking the same questions, but never giving him any answers nor providing any relief. The frequent visits to office, clinic, and hospital, and the dreary time spent waiting in these places, would prevent him from working even if he were able, and drain him emotionally as well as physically (and in some cases, financially). He distrusts the doctors, and resents all the useless tests and appointments, but fears to express these feelings because, who knows? Maybe something will turn up, or someone will have an answer.

Moreover, all the questions and examinations force the patient to notice and think about his symptoms more than he ever has before. His pain is insistent enough, but now he notices all the other bodily feelings that previously went unnoticed: the twinges, itches, tinglings, and aches. Noticing and paying attention to them magnifies them, and soon they are more frequent and more noticeable, and soon the patient begins to answer more doctors' questions affirmatively, and then even volunteers the information about these sensations as new symptoms which bother him. Partly this is because he is worried about them, as a sign that his illness is spreading or getting worse, and partly because he is hopeful that the new information will somehow help the doctors find something that can be treated and so relieve his suffering.

As time goes on, and the patient feels more wretched and desperate, he begins to cast about for some magical cure. He hears about cases similar to his who were treated successfully, or he reads something about a new clinic or treatment technique, and soon he is seeking out a hypnotist, an acupuncturist, or an evangelical preacher. Their treatments may help for a while, but then the pain returns, and the patient returns to his doctor asking for stronger analgesics or surgical relief.

A MINORITY GROUP

The description just given is a composite of a great many patients' experiences, and so may not fit any one individual. It seems to apply, more or less aptly, to the majority of patients who seek help from doctors for their chronic pain problem. However, there is a small minority of patients who do not permit themselves to succumb to this pattern and so are not often seen by doctors. They hurt just as badly as the others, but do not persist in seeking relief. They seem too busy, too engaged in their world to have much time for doctors. They say, "Doctor, if you can do something for this pain, that's fine. And if you can't—that's fine too—I'll just live with it."

Their analysis of medications seems more analytical than most of the other patients', less colored by wishful thinking or desperation. They say, "Doctor, those pills don't do that much for my pain, and they seem to cloud my mind. I'm going to stop taking them."

They seem to enjoy working. If they are unable to perform at their former job, they find something else that they can do, sometimes going to school for retraining. If they accept disability compensation, which is rare, it is only for a brief interim period. They seem proud of their independence and ability to overcome their handicaps, but the motivation seems to be the enjoyment of accomplishment rather than the need to prove anything to others. They say, "I just can't lie around and do nothing. I have to keep busy."

As these patients are a small proportion of those in chronic pain, and do not see doctors or come to hospitals as often, we can be less sure of their experiences as compared with the others. But we have some clues, from the things they say, that their lives and attitudes are quite different.

"When I was first hurt I used to get a lot of sympathy and pity from the nurses and volunteers in the hospital. I used to eat it up, and really enjoyed feeling sorry for myself. Then I got tired of the whole thing. I figured it wasn't getting me anywhere, so I got out of the hospital and took a job and started going to school at night."

"I'm a nut about gardening. I work in my garden about four or five hours a day. I can't stand or walk so I kind of sit and drag myself along, and I can do everything I used to do. I don't know what I'd do if I couldn't take care of my plants."

"You've got to fight the pain, you can't give in to it."

"You have to do something, anything just to get started, and then you find out what you like and do that. If you stop, you lose ground, and your pain actually gets worse."

"I've been living with this thing for 17 years now, and I'd like to get some relief. My doctor heard about this place and thought I should come here because you have some new treatments or something. Well I hope I'm not being too crude, but I don't want to waste your time and mine, and if you don't think you can help my case just tell me and we'll call it quits. I don't want to take too much time away from my family."

These patients clearly begrudge any time away from their usual daily routines, and unlike the others, they are not afraid to express this attitude. They insist on a more businesslike relationship with doctors than that of beseecher and besought; if the doctors don't have what the patients want, then the patients drop the matter, rather than continue shopping.

There is also, clearly, a strong defense of the boundaries of the subjective world. The patients fight to maintain their interests and relationships with family, friends, job, and hobbies. They refuse to permit their pain to interfere with any of this. Some, in fact, have let themselves withdraw, only to find that they became worse, so they fought back to reestablish the wider boundaries.

What we know about the subjective experiences of chronic pain patients can now help us to appreciate more formal studies of the effects of chronic pain.

III

Psychological Effects of Chronic Pain

From what we have been able to learn of the pain patient's experience, it seems to change him in significant ways. His perception of the world, his relationship with others, his preoccupations, and his activities all seem to alter rather markedly.

In order to determine if this is indeed the case, and if so, to what extent this is, we need to have some objective data with which to confirm these subjective impressions. The ideal situation, of course, would be to have objective personality profiles of a large group of patients before they become afflicted with chronic pain, and then obtain similar profiles at periodic intervals thereafter. This would permit a quantitative evaluation of the impact of pain on the individuals enduring it. However, except for certain fortuitous cases, this information is seldom available.

Systematic studies of pain patients are hard to come by. There are many reports of patients with complaints of pain, but these are usually of the sort which seek to determine, for example, what percentage of those who complain of headaches or pelvic pain have psychological problems; or there are psychological profiles of patients who complain of some pain problem, are found not to have any detectable organic pathology, and are referred for psychiatric evaluation. Such reports are relatively common and are reviewed by Merskey and Spear (53); however, they are of little help to us in our present inquiry. We seek to know precisely what organically caused pain does to people, so that we can help them effectively.

A few recent studies, primarily by British investigators, contain information that is relevant. Although the studies were designed for different purposes than to answer the question we have raised, they do provide objective data on patients with chronic pain referrable to physical causes.

Bond and Pearson (9) reported on 52 women hospitalized with advanced cancer of the cervix. They were tested with the Eysenck Personality Inventory; their lower and upper pain thresholds were measured; they expressed their level of pain numerically; and a record was made of their requests for analgesics and the medications given. Personality scores were compared with those of a group of women medical patients without pain, and a group of normal housewives was used for further comparison. Pain thresholds were also compared with the medical patient group.

Of all this information, we are primarily interested in the personality scores of the cancer patients. The Eysenck Personality Inventory yields two scores, one for Neuroticism, the other for Extraversion. On neither of these did the cancer patients differ significantly from the housewives comprising the standardization group.

However, Bond and Pearson found that the 52 cancer patients could be divided into three groups: 13 women without pain, and who therefore did not receive analgesics; 17 women with pain, who did not, however, receive analgesics; and 22 women with pain who did receive analgesics. These three subgroups had different personality scores, as shown in Table 1. The authors consider that the Neuroticism scores may be related to levels of arousal, or sensitivity to stimuli (including pain), and that Extraversion scores may be related to the readiness to communicate freely or to complain; extraverts are also said to have high thresholds.

Thus, as can be seen in Table 3.1, the cancer patients without pain had low Neuroticism scores, and were quite outgoing. Those with pain were more neurotic. These more neurotic women differed in whether or not they asked for and received analgesics; the introverted women did not receive analgesics, whereas the extraverted ones did.

Bond and Pearson, although conservative in the interpretation of their data, imply that these preexisting personality traits determine to some extent whether the patients experience pain and express this experience. Of course, it is possible

TABLE 3.1 Neuroticism and Extraversion Scores of Women Cancer Patients[a]

Group	Neuroticism	Extraversion
No pain, no analgesics (*N* = 13)	Low	High
Pain, no analgesics (*N* = 17)	High	Low
Pain, received analgesics (*N* = 22)	High	High

[a] Summarized from Bond and Pearson (9), used by permission of Microforms International Marketing Corp., exclusive copyright lessee of Pergamon Press journal back files.

too that the high Neuroticism scores are the *result* of being in pain, rather than a cause (or part of the cause) of the pain experience. Unfortunately, we have no information as to how long the women had been ill, or to the duration of the pain experience, nor do we know whether the subgroups differed in this respect.

In a further report on these patients, Bond (8) compared the results of the Eysenck Personality Inventory with other test data from the Cornell Medical Index and Whiteley Index of Hypochondriasis. The results of the latter two tests for the three subgroups of patients are summarized in Table 3.2.

TABLE 3.2 Symptoms and Hypochondriasis Scores of Women Cancer Patients[a]

Group	Cornell Medical Index	Whiteley Index of Hypochondriasis
No pain, no analgesics ($N = 13$)	Low	Low
Pain, no analgesics ($N = 17$)	High	High
Pain, received analgesics ($N = 22$)	High	High

[a] Summarized from Bond (8) used by permission of M. R. Bond and the *British Journal of Psychiatry.*

The Cornell Medical Index is made up of a checklist of both physical and emotional symptoms experienced in the past and present; high scores are considered indicative of emotional disturbance. It can be seen that the patients with pain are high in this regard, supporting the previous findings from the Eysenck Personality Inventory.

The Whiteley Index of Hypochondriasis was devised by Pilowsky (58) and measures (a) bodily preoccupation, (b) disease phobia which the patient seeks to deny, and (c) a conviction of disease which does not respond to reassurance, and which at times may be considered psychotic. We shall be considering this test in some detail in a later chapter, but it is interesting to note here that the women cancer patients with pain scored high on these tests, and in all three categories, obtained scores comparable to hypochondriacal psychiatric patients among comparison groups. In contrast, the women cancer patients without pain had low scores, comparable to those of normal subjects, and these fell in the category of "disease phobia which the patient seeks to deny."

Bond presents evidence to support his contention that these personality factors influence the experience and expression of pain. Again, it may be the other way around, because correlation is no index of causation, and in the absence of longitudinal data from a prospective study we cannot be certain. However, the two studies so far do show that, in a group of patients of the same sex, disease, and site of lesion, pain is associated with neuroticism and an increased awareness of physical and emotional symptoms, whereas the absence of pain is associated with the opposite.

Woodforde and Merskey (93) administered the Middlesex Hospital Questionnaire and the Eysenck Personality Inventory to 43 patients with chronic pain. It is not stated what duration of time is meant by "chronic," but from the diseases (nonmalignant) represented (94), a minimum of several months is probable. Of these 43 patients, 27 had pain due to organic disease, and 16 were determined to have psychogenic pain. The group is biased in that all were referred for psychiatric consultation, but many of the organic pain patients were referred only for advice on the treatment of their pain.

The Middlesex Hospital Questionnaire gives scores for a number of neurotic traits, such as anxiety, phobia, obsessionality, somatic preoccupation, etc. On all these scales, the pain patients scored higher than normals, and obtained scores comparable to those of psychiatric outpatients. There were no significant differences between those with organic lesions and those with psychological diseases.

On the Eysenck Personality Inventory, also, the pain patients had significantly higher neuroticism scores than normals, again comparable to psychiatric outpatients, and were more introverted than normals; there were no differences between the two subgroups of pain patients. In addition, the male organic pain patients obtained high "Lie" scores, reflecting a socially desirable test-taking attitude (trying to appear healthy), a finding which Bond (8) had also noted in all three of his subgroups of women cancer patients.

Woodforde and Merskey conclude that the effect of chronic pain is to cause emotional disturbance. They argue that although there is evidence of neuroticism causing psychogenic pain, there is none suggesting that organic pain is more often associated with certain personality types. They also feel that there were no particularly great psychological stresses exacerbating the organic pain in their patients. Once again, this argument is inferential, but it is clear that chronic pain and neuroticism appear to be associated. If it is assumed by definition that the group with chronic pain not due to organic causes is neurotic, and this is confirmed by the psychological test scores, then the similar scores of the patients with organic lesions suggests that they are indistinguishable from the psychiatric group in this respect.

In another report, Woodforde and Merskey (94) tested these patients' pain levels using four different techniques. On these tasks, too, the groups did not differ.

A different way of looking at the effect of pain, when the longitudinal approach is impractical, is to employ the cross-sectional approach, that is, to compare different groups of patients at various stages of their illness. A first attempt at this was made by Sternbach *et al.* (80), who examined 117 low-back patients seen consecutively in an orthopedic low-back clinic. Of this group, 19 had pain for less than 6 months and were considered to be "acute;" 98 had pain for 6 months or more, and were considered "chronic." These patients were tested on the Minnesota Multiphasic Personality Inventory (MMPI), and their profiles are shown in Fig. 3.

The average score for the normal population is defined as 50, and scores two or more standard deviations above the mean (70 and higher) are considered to be clinically significant. In examining the profiles in Fig. 3, it is quite apparent that the two groups differ significantly on the first three scales, which are Hypochondriasis, Depression, and Hysteria. These three comprise the so-called "neurotic triad," and those with chronic pain obtain clinically significant scores on these scales, whereas those with acute pain are within normal limits on all scales.

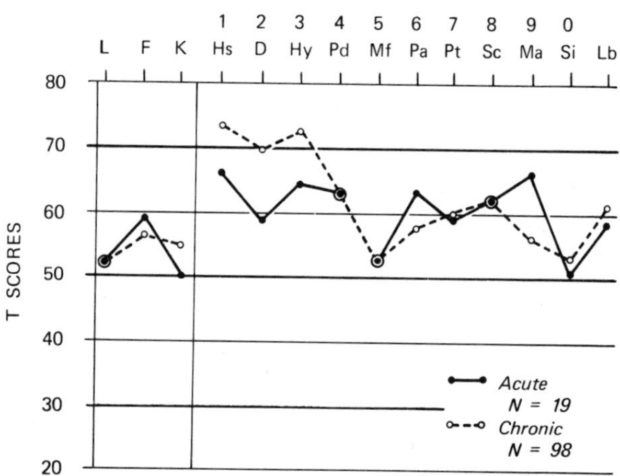

Fig. 3. Comparison of profiles of 19 acute low back patients and 98 chronic low back patients. Scales 1, 2, 3, and 9 are significantly different for the two groups. (After Sternbach *et al.*, 1973, reproduced by permission of *Psychosomatics.*)

Clinical interpretation of these profiles, based on extensive research (19), permits our making certain inferences. If we think of the acute patients as those who will, with the passage of time, become chronic patients, we can examine this profile for tendencies which will predict such results.

There is a clear trend toward a psychophysiological reaction in the acute patients, shown by the relative relationships of the first three scales: higher scores on Hypochondriasis (scale 1) and Hysteria (scale 3) and a lower score on Depression (scale 2). This is so common a finding that it is called the "psychosomatic-V." It reflects a somatic preoccupation, and a tendency to deny emotional disturbance, so that, in psychodynamic jargon, somatization serves to bind the affect, and so depression is not apparent. In other words, the patients focus on their low-back pain to avoid the awareness of being depressed.

However, there also seems to be a considerable amount of reaction–formation to the latent depression. This is shown to some extent by the agitation which is reflected in the Psychopathic (scale 4) and Paranoid (scale 6) elevations, but even more by the Mania (scale 9) score, which also differentiates the two groups at a statistically significant level.

Looking next at the profile of the chronic patients, on the assumption that it evolved from a pattern like that of the acute patients, we can see that the defense mechanisms of somatization and hypomanic reaction–formation have failed. There is now much greater somatic concern, and a significant amount of depression with no compensatory hypomania.

Of course it is only speculation that the patients with chronic pain formerly had more normal-looking psychological profiles, but it is not an unreasonable inference. Clinical impression tends to support this view, in that the life histories of chronic pain patients show that most of them functioned quite adequately, at home, at work, and in social situations, prior to the disease or injury that resulted in persistent pain. It is at least probable that these patients would have obtained a normal composite profile prior to their affliction, and that after a few months their scores would have looked like those of the acute patients, intermediate between the normal and chronic profiles.

These few studies, on rather different populations and using different measuring instruments, tend to confirm the impressions gained from patients' descriptions of their experiences. The patients are emotionally disturbed; the form of this disturbance is neurotic; the neurotic characteristics consist of hypochondriasis and depression. In the patients' terms, they become preoccupied with their symptoms to the exclusion of almost everything else, and feel quite hopeless about their condition. Now that we have evidence that their reaction to chronic pain is not just their imagination, but is sufficiently marked to be measurable, it may be instructive to consider an illustrative case history.

CASE ILLUSTRATION 1

Mrs. B. D. is a 50-year-old married mother of two with a 5-year history of low-back and left-leg pain which has persisted despite a discectomy and laminectomy. She is seen for psychological evaluation as part of a total workup considering the possibilities of a rhizotomy or the implantation of a dorsal column stimulator.

Relevant History. The patient has an older brother and sister still living in the Midwest, and two much younger brothers in this area. The patient's father (age 89) and mother (age 79) also live here. They have recently been in cardiac intensive care units, and for the past year the patient has performed heroic nursing tasks for them in her home, despite her limitations. The job fell to her since her children are grown, whereas her younger brothers still have children at home. The patient's daughter, age 28, is happily married and about to have her fourth child. The son, age 26, is also married and just had a third child.

The patient's son, son-in-law, and husband (age 53) are all store or operations managers for big discount chains. Her husband just quit his job and is considering other possibilities, one of which would take them to the Midwest next year. The patient denies any preference for staying or leaving here (they have been here 14 years), saying she is happy if her husband is.

The pain has prevented her from doing much of her housework, and she feels that this is her job. For 2 years, after her children married and before her accident, she kept house, but also accompanied her husband on his frequent business trips. She is now limited in her ability to drive, and she can no longer take camping trips, fish from their boat, or walk in the woods. She also finds that by the end of the day, her thinking is clouded because of the analgesics (APC with codeine, two taken four times daily). She finds herself generally irritable and tense, and stays up until 1:00 AM in order to be exhausted when she gets to bed. She sleeps through the night until about 7:30 or 8:00 AM. Although she smokes two to three packs of cigarettes a day, it is not due to the pain, but has been a habit all her adult life, which she says is "because I'm highstrung."

Whenever she described her pain, or the effect it has had on her, Mrs. D's lips quivered, and she was obviously fighting tears. Yet, despite her obvious discomfort, and abstention from her usual analgesics in order to be mentally clear for the interview, she managed to remain seated for 2½ hours of interviewing and testing, and she got up without much difficulty.

Test Findings. On the Health Index, Mrs. D. endorsed very few items. She apparently does not consider herself an invalid, is not manifestly depressed, is not preoccupied with pain, nor does she play pain games with doctors.

Mrs. D. estimates the usual severity of her clinical pain (left hip and posterior left knee) at about 65 on a scale of 0 to 100. This is in the moderate to severe range. On the arm ischemic pain test, this usual intensity was matched at 3 min 35 sec, and her maximum tolerance was reached in 6 min 5 sec. Thus her clinical pain is 59%, of her tolerance on this test, and this is in good agreement with her estimate of 65.

Her MMPI profile shows a significant degree of "faking psychological health" with defensiveness and evasiveness, causing her to receive somewhat reduced scores on the clinical scales, and she makes extensive use of the defense mechanism of denial (Fig. 4). With moderate elevations on the hypochondriasis and hysteria scales, but no signs of depression or anxiety, she has a strong potential for hysterical–conversion reactions. Her defensiveness was also marked

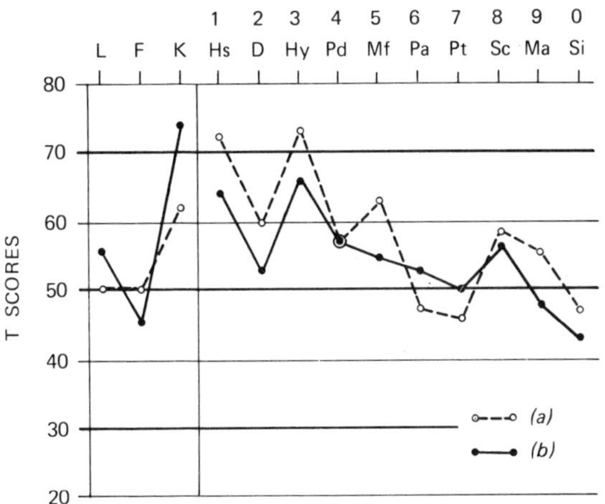

Fig. 4. MMPI profiles of patient B.D., (a) 10 mo prior to the interview (b) consultation.

on an MMPI take 10 months ago, though not so extreme as it is now, and as a consequence her tendency to somatization reaction appeared more clearly then.

By a "somatization reaction" in this patient, we are referring to the use of a physical symptom to avoid awareness of threatening affect. Mrs. D. seems to be focusing on her pain in a successful attempt to avoid a reactive depression to her limitations.

Discussion. This patient seems to be a successful and happy housewife. There are no apparent gains for her in this situation, no payoff for being ill. She seems to have good relationships with her parents, husband, children, and grandchildren. Her pain test is straightforward and clear and in good agreement with her estimate of the pain severity, so she is an accurate reporter of her pain.

Mrs. D. has an hysterical personality type that is essentially within normal limits. She has had ample opportunity to use this disease to manipulate others, but she has not; to abuse drugs, but has not. She is still able to use her defense mechanism of denial to ward off a reactive depression. The MMPI ego-strength score is high, incidentally, confirming what is obvious from her life-style.

Diagnostic Impression. Hysterical personality, mild (301.56), with denial of latent depression and invalid reactions.

Recommendation. An excellent candidate for a surgical procedure, unlikely to sabotage surgical pain relief with psychological problems.

IV

Psychogenic Pain

Now it will be useful, for purposes of comparison, to examine the characteristics of those whose pain is of psychological origin, even though our chief interest lies with those having physically caused pain. Our hope is that information about one group will help our understanding of the other. First, however, we must avoid some misunderstandings.

By the term "psychogenic pain" we do not mean to imply psychological "pain" such as suffering or grieving. These are unpleasant experiences but are not associated with tissue damage nor described in terms of tissue damage.

Neither do we mean to imply that psychogenic pain is experienced differently from that arising from physical disease or injury. There are some authors who have said this, but on no basis of evidence whatever except their assertion that such pain must be "imaginary" or "painless pain."

In my personal experience, having experienced both, psychogenic and somatogenic pain feel the same; this is supported by the descriptions given by patients in both groups. In fact, it is precisely because patients are so consistently similar in their descriptions of their experiences that so much care is taken by clinicians to differentiate psychogenic and somatogenic pain, a task which is frequently very difficult. Like effects can certainly arise from dissimilar causes.

Another point, which needs clarification, has to do with the dualism with which we view ourselves. This is apparently peculiar to our Western society (e.g., 24), and is not very helpful in our understanding of phenomenon such as the experience of pain. Elsewhere (70,71) I have pointed out that, following the suggestions of Szasz (82), we can do better by not insisting on classifying a pain as psychogenic or somatogenic, but rather by seeing whether a description of causes in psychological or physical languages is more helpful. Merskey and Spear (53) independently advanced the same view.

"Psychogenic" is a statement of a causative relationship, and rather than become entangled in a discussion of how an experience of physical sensations can arise from mental events, it is, in our view, better to say that we are simply describing the experience in the language of psychology or, alternatively, in the language of physiology. Graham (29) has made a persuasive case for this view, which he calls "linguistic parallelism," applied to a spectrum of the so-called psychosomatic disorders.

This view has quite practical advantages in dealing with patients in pain. Rather than trying to decide whether a particular patient *has* psychogenic *or* somatogenic pain, a frequently impossible decision to make, as it implies two different states, it is much more helpful to describe his problem in psychological *and* physical terms and pursue the indicated treatments in parallel. We will describe this procedure in greater detail in a later chapter.

It is unfortunate that our customary way of thinking makes it difficult to express this approach in an apt phrase. Current usage favors the term "psychogenic," which means, "due to psychological causes." In deference to custom we will continue to use the term, but we are explicit in stating that we mean, "pain which is better described and understood in psychological than in physical language." In practice, this usually means that an adequate physical explanation for the pain experience cannot be given, whereas an adequate explanation in psychological terms can be given.

This approach honors the integrity of the patient's pain experience. It does not imply, as does the traditional view, that he is "imagining" his pain, or that it is not real, or that it is not really pain. That is, description in parallel languages assumes what clinical experience in fact suggests, that there is a single phenomenon—pain—and not two phenomena—"painful pain" and "painless pain."

Accordingly, in this chapter particularly (but also elsewhere in this book), whenever the term "psychogenic pain" is used, it refers to *pain which is better understood in psychological than in physical language.* Similarly, psychogenic pain patients are those whose experience of pain is less adequately explained in physical terms than in psychological terms. Psychogenic pain patients do *not* hurt less, or differently, than the somatogenic pain patients whose experience is more adequately explainable in physical terms. The study by Woodforde and Merskey (94) cited in the previous chapter supports clinical experience that there seems to be little if any difference in the pain experiences of psychogenic and somatogenic pain patients.

Let us now turn to the studies of psychogenic pain patients. These patients are usually studied by psychiatrists and psychologists because numbers of them are referred by physicians and surgeons who cannot find adequate physical explanations for the pain complaints. Such a series was reported by Woodforde and Merskey (93), and as noted in the previous chapter, there were no significant differences in psychological test scores between the two patient groups (psychogenic and somatogenic).

Pilling *et al.* (57) examined data of 562 patients seen in consultation at Mayo Clinic. Of 221 males, 65 had pain and 156 did not, and of 341 females, 117 had pain and 224 did not. Thus the comparison was essentially between a presumed psychogenic pain group and a presumed psychosomatic group (other physical symptoms than pain). The examination consisted of a clinical interview, information recorded on a sixty-three-item checklist, and the results from the Minnesota Multiphasic Personality Inventory. The authors' psychiatric evaluations indicated that depression was less frequent in the patients with pain than in those without pain, while hypochondriasis was more frequent in those with pain than in those without pain. The test profiles tended to support this observation, as shown in Fig. 5.

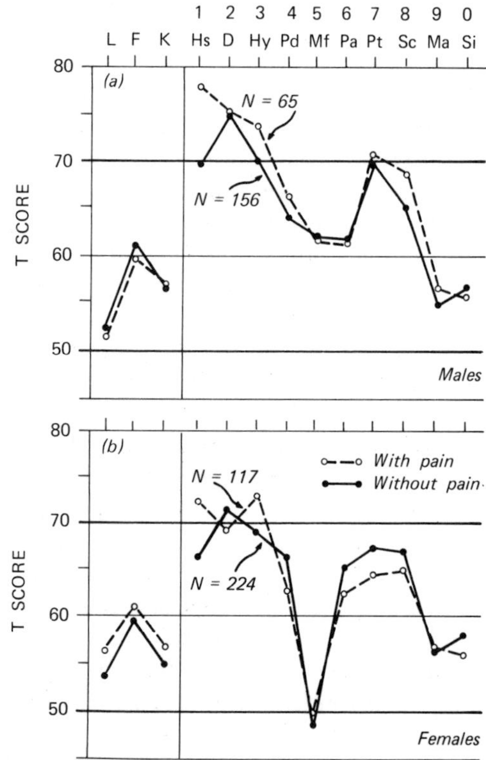

Fig. 5. MMPI profiles of men (a) and women (b) with and without pain, referred for psychiatric consultation. (After Pilling *et al.*, 1967, reproduced by permission of *Canadian Medical Association Journal.*)

Examination of these profiles shows that all the patients have neurotic patterns, that hypochondriasis and depression are significant features of this pattern, and that the pain patients have significantly more hypochondriasis than those with physical symptoms other than pain. The authors conclude, on the basis of their interviews and the test results, that pain may be substituted for feelings of anxiety and depression, in that pain as a symptom may be less distressing than these other feelings.

A similar finding in a homogeneous patient group was reported by Castelnuovo-Tedesco and Krout (15). They examined three groups of women with gynecological problems. Group A consisted of 40 women of lower socioeconomic class *with* chronic (5 months or more) pelvic pain; 25 had demonstrable organic pelvic pathology, 15 did not. Group B consisted of 27 women from the same lower socioeconomic class, with organic pelvic pathology but *without* chronic pelvic pain. Group C consisted of 25 women from a lower middle-class setting with complaints of chronic pelvic pain.

The authors found that regardless of the presence or absence of organic pain pathology, pelvic pain patients showed considerable clinical psychopathology—predominantly character disorders with schizoid features. The Minnesota Multiphasic Personality Inventory profiles showed that Groups A and C (pelvic pain) demonstrated more psychopathology than did Group B (pelvic pathology without pain). These results are shown in Fig. 6.

In this study, scores are not as elevated as in previously reported populations, but the profiles are somewhat similar. Groups A and C have higher scores on the Hypochondriasis and Hysteria scales, suggesting to the authors that these

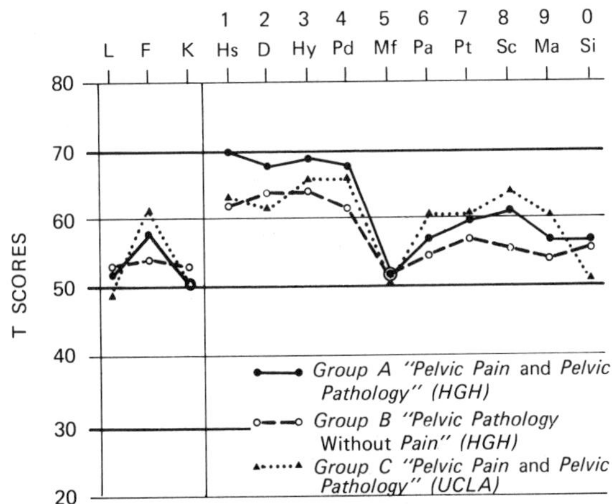

Fig. 6. MMPI profiles of three groups of gynecological patients. (After Castelnuovo-Tedesco and Krout, 1970, reproduced by permission of *International Journal of Psychiatry in Medicine*, published by Baywood Publishing Co.)

patients make greater use of somatization, denial, and repression as defenses. In contrast, Group B has Depression scores higher than its own scores on Hypochondriasis and Hysteria, indicating that these patients experience and show more depression than do those with pain. These findings tend to support the suggestion of Pilling *et al.* (57) that pain may be substituted for an unpleasant affect like depression. The two groups of women with pain show more hypochondriacal concerns relative to their depression, while the reverse is true for the women without pain.

Merskey (49,50) examined 100 psychiatric patients with pain complaints of more than 3-months duration, and compared them with 65 patients without pain. He found that there was a greater percentage of neurotic conditions, especially hysteria, among the pain patients. He failed to find increased scores for Neuroticism on the Maudsley Personality Inventory, and in a later report (51) confirmed that, unlike reports of patients with organic pain, or those medical patients with psychogenic pain (93), the psychiatric patients obtained scores comparable to those for normals. Patients already in a psychiatric setting, presumably differ from those in a medical setting, and the patients studied by Merskey may well have been masking their neurotic symptoms by focusing on their pain, thus obtaining scores closer to that of normals.

Sternbach *et al.* (80), in the study of consecutive admissions to a low-back clinic cited in the previous chapter, compared the MMPI profiles of two groups of patients, those with physical findings on examination, and those without such findings. The term positive physical findings refers to results of orthopedic examination including muscle atrophy, diminished sensation, decreased deep tendon reflexes, positive straight leg raising, and the like, supported by x-ray examination and, in some instances, a myelogram. These two groups, 81 people with findings and 36 people with no findings, are compared in Fig. 7.

The apparent difference between the groups on the Depression scale is not statistically significant, while the small difference on the Manic scale just barely reaches significance. The Low-Back scale, originally designed to distinguish between "functional" and "organic" low backs, does not do so here. Essentially, the profiles of the two groups are the same. The patients with no findings, presumably psychogenic pain patients, are as hypochondriacal and depressed as those with somatogenic pain. This finding is similar to that reported by Woodforde and Merskey (93) comparing mixed pain syndromes of organic and psychiatric origin.

There is a great number of similar studies, examining series of patients with headaches, chest pains, etc., and the few studies which have been cited here are quite representative. Further review would only be repetitious. The major point, which can be made with some certainty, is that those people with psychogenic pain tend to be neurotic, and in this respect do not differ much from those with chronic pain of organic origin.

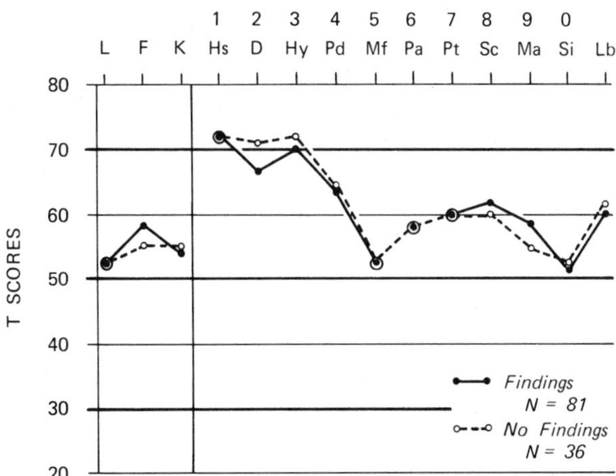

Fig. 7. Comparison of MMPI profiles of low back pain patients with and without physical findings. (After Sternbach *et al.*, 1973, reproduced by permission of *Psychosomatics.*)

The test scores that we have shown are of limited usefulness in that they categorize, but they tell us little about how psychogenic pain patients become neurotic. To obtain this kind of information we must turn to reports of extended psychiatric interviews. Generally, these come from psychodynamically (psychoanalytically) oriented sources.

PSYCHODYNAMIC INVESTIGATIONS

An extensive clinical–theoretical report has been provided by Engel (23), who summarizes the characteristics of "pain-prone patients." These are individuals who repeatedly suffer painful disability, with or without detectable physical lesions. Almost always, according to Engel, these patients have excessive guilt feelings, conscious or unconscious, and the experience of pain serves as punishment which serves to relieve these guilt feelings. Such patients repeatedly get themselves into situations or relationships in which they are hurt and defeated, and this is when their health is best. Conversely, when their life situation improves, they suffer again (or more) from pain. They are thus intolerant of success.

These patients usually were reared in a family situation in which aggression and pain figured prominently. Either the patients experienced frequent abuse, thus learning that painful attention meant that the parents cared (as other children learn to value affection), or else distant parents showed concern only when the patients were sick or hurt. In any event, a pattern of suffering was usually established in childhood.

In adolescence and adulthood, specific incidents typically initiate or exacerbate the pain states. These may be: some form of success which threatens the role of suffering person, a real or threatened loss, or the arousal of strong and forbidden feelings (usually sexual or aggressive ones) which must be controlled. The experience of pain serves to sabotage impending success, and reaffirms the suffering role. It also serves to punish the individual for his unacceptable hostile, sexual, or dependent impulses, as he may have been punished for the expression of these in childhood.

In the case of a loss of someone important to the patient, the pain may be experienced as part of the mechanism of identification, in which the patient identifies with that person as a child identifies with a parent. The pain is usually one that the patient experienced when in conflict with that person, or one that the person had or the patient imagines he had. Thus the pain seems a way of keeping the important person "alive" through the identification process.

Szasz (82) proposes a general psychoanalytic theory of pain. His view is that pain results from the perception of a threat to the integrity of the body. The threat may be real or imagined; what is necessary for pain is the perception of it. This accounts for the instances of injury without pain, as well as the instances of pain without injury. Whether or not the pain is classified as "real" or "imaginary" depends on whether an observer finds objective evidence of the threat. Usually that decision is made by a physician looking for signs of physical injury.

Szasz states that the body is treated as an "object" by the ego, which is separate from it. That is, the ego values the body in the same way it values important other persons (also termed "objects" in psychoanalysis). The ego thus experiences anxiety and pain when an important part or body function is lost. This constitutes the first level of meaning of pain, pain as a symptom.

A second level of meaning is that of communication, in which pain is a form of interpersonal behavior, used as a means of soliciting help. In the usual case, the first two levels—subjective symptom and request for aid—are the forms of pain behavior presented to the doctor. A third level of meaning, symbolic, is less well defined but presumably involves such various forms of interpersonal manipulations as passive–aggressive behavior via pain complaints, and similar secondary gains. These and other forms of pain behavior will be discussed in a later chapter.

The gist of these psychodynamic descriptions is that, given an exposure to a certain form of abusiveness in childhood, individuals adopt a life-style in which suffering is a key factor. Certain precipitating experiences can initiate or exacerbate pain states in these predisposed persons. Such a model describes both

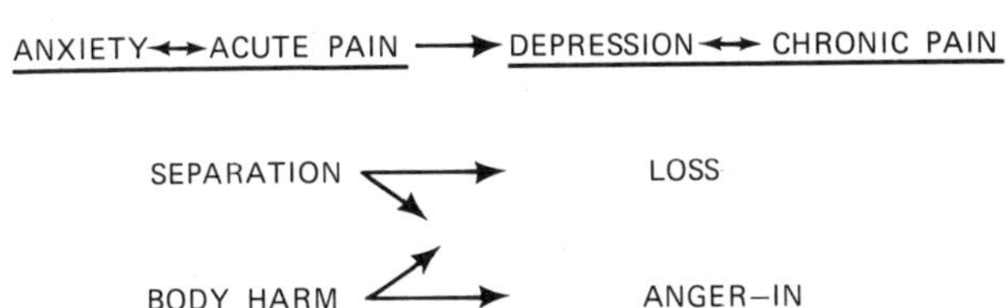

Fig. 8. The development of chronic pain from acute pain.

acute and recurrent episodes of psychogenic pain, and also the chronic or persistent pain case. This can be represented schematically as in Fig. 8.

The affect which we historically associate with experiences of acute pain is anxiety. Anxiety is either that type concerning a threatened separation from an important person, as in their withdrawal of love, or that type concerning a threatened injury, as occurs with punishment. Anxiety, therefore, is the affect that occurs when we anticipate what might happen.

When what is feared actually does come to pass, we feel grief, or we feel punished, and these are the basic causes of depression. Unresolved grief, and intropunitive anger, are the major dynamic processes underlying reactive depression, and it is this depression which we find associated with chronic pain.

The above is a brief synopsis of extensive writings, and is meant to be only an outline. What is interesting is that certain hypotheses can be generated from this psychodynamic model and tested against objective findings.

For example, if the hypothesis about chronicity is correct, we would expect to find a significant association with depression. We have already reviewed a number of studies which show this to be the case. The clinical observations of Engel that the pain-prone patients have a high incidence of painful injuries and operations and tend to be resentful and hostile persons (a sign of their intropunitive anger), has also been borne out by objective studies reviewed by Merskey and Spear (53). Tinling and Klein (86) also reported on a series of men with chronic psychogenic pain, whose anger was only partly sublimated by solitary hunting and driving "hot rods."

The prediction that pain serves partly to relieve guilt feelings is supported by the findings of Pilling *et al.* (57), and by Castelnuovo-Tedesco and Krout (15), which show relatively lower depression scores in patients with pain complaints as compared with control patients without pain complaints.

In general as Merskey and Spear (53) observed, the clinical descriptions made by psychodynamically oriented psychiatrists, and the psychoanalytic inferences about the underlying mechanisms, seem to be supported where objective data can be obtained. Psychogenic pain patients, like those who have had organically caused pain for some time, seem to be neurotically depressed and hypochondriacal. They appear to have gotten that way because they were raised in a setting where pain and suffering were associated with attention (as a substitute for normal affection), and later pain episodes are easily precipitated by loss, or by intropunitive anger for unwanted success or feelings of aggression, sexuality, or dependency.

As the two groups of pain patients seem to have in common the features of hypochondriasis and depression, we will examine these in greater detail in order better to understand pain patients, but first we will consider an illustrative case history.

CASE ILLUSTRATION 2

Mr. A. V. is a 53-year-old male who is seen because of complaints of low-back and right-leg pain of $2\frac{1}{2}$-years duration. This began with a train accident in July 1970, and was exacerbated by a more serious train accident in September 1971. Orthopedic and neurological examinations are negative.

Interview. Mr. V. appears relaxed and friendly and appropriately concerned about his condition. He relates a good deal of bitterness against the railroad company for which he works as a conductor. He feels he has served them well and faithfully for 32 years, and has now been treated badly by them in that they have failed to provide adequate medical referral and have insisted on his returning to work. He has retained lawyers to get his lost back wages and disability or pension payments. He is here at his own expense, because his daughter works here as a nurse and assures him he can get proper evaluation and treatment. In heavy Southern "country boy" accents, he attempts to flatter us for our expertness, and minimizes the role of the pending litigation in perpetuating his pain. He states he is leery of the surgery recommended by doctors he was sent to by lawyers. He has been taking six to eight Darvon per day.

Test Findings. On the Health Index, there was no significant number of items endorsed in the categories of chronic invalidism, manifest depression, or playing pain games with doctors, and only a moderate amount of preoccupation with pain.

Mr. V. estimates his usual pain severity as 40 on a scale of 0–100, which is in the slight to moderate range. On the submaximum effort tourniquet technique for arm ischemic pain, his usual clinical pain was matched in severity at 25 sec, and his maximum tolerance was reached in 2 min 0 sec. Thus his usual pain is 21% of tolerance, which is slight, and his estimate is somewhat exaggerated.

The MMPI shows some feelings of helplessness and a willingness to admit to difficulties with less than the normal amounts of defensiveness (Fig. 9). This is

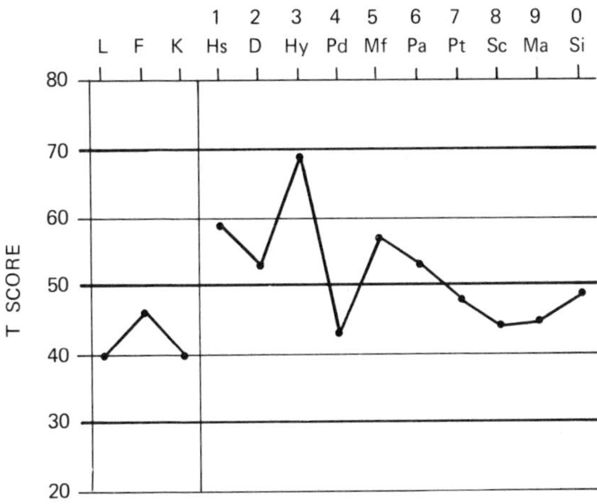

Fig. 9. MMPI profile of patient A.V.

probably associated with an inability to cope with his disability. Despite this, all clinical scales are essentially within normal limits. The profile interpretation is that of a person with rather strong dependency needs, a tendency to deny emotional problems, and thus a potential for developing conversion symptoms or a "functional overlay" when the needs are not met.

Discussion. Mr. V. was presented with a summary of all findings: that the neurosurgeon could not find evidence of neurological deficit on examination or x-ray; that the pain seemed not to be great; and that he probably had some muscle damage which should have healed, but that emotional problems were making the pain persist.

With some embarrassment Mr. V. confessed to a great fear of working on the trains following the last serious accident. He tried to overcome this when he worked again from April to November 1972, but could not. As evidence that he was not abnormal in this reaction, he noted that his partner who only received a bump in the accident is similarly afraid, and has taken to drinking heavily to force himself to work. Mr. V. has been through many derailments and minor accidents, but this last serious one has caused him, apparently, to lose his nerve. As he would not normally admit this fear to himself, it seems that his continued back pain is a substitute which is more honorable for him: "It is not that I'm afraid to work, it is this bad back which prevents me."

Mr. V. also admitted to being impotent since the last accident, and suggested himself that this was probably "mental." This also suggests that the impact of the accident was quite severe, in that the patient, with his fear, feels quite helpless and stripped of his manhood and dignity.

In discussing this problem, and possible solutions, with the patient, he felt he could not overcome this fear, knowing as he does the railroads' failure to correct defective equipment, etc. He cannot move to an inside job because he loses all seniority if he does and thus is likely to be fired. He thinks that his best solution may be to take his pension and try to find other work.

Formulation and Diagnostic Impression. The persistent pain is a legitimate ticket out of an intolerable situation for the patient who is now too frightened to work on the trains and who cannot admit to himself how frightened he is. This situation has been compounded by his dependency needs. He has been loyal to the company for 32 years, but when he became hurt he did not receive the paternal benevolence he expected, and instead was met with harsh demands. Thus, he has been forced into a sick role to satisfy these needs. Accordingly, the appropriate diagnoses seem to be:

1. Psychophysiological musculoskeletal disorder (305.16);
2. adjustment reaction of adulthood, post-traumatic neurosis (307.36).

Recommendation. The two reasonable alternatives for Mr. V. are, apparently, behavior therapy for desensitization of his phobia, or a change of jobs. The latter seems more realistic, because the phobia is not entirely conscious and he continues to have physical symptoms; these did not diminish when the patient returned to work for 7 months. Mr. V. seemed to prefer the solution of settling with the company as soon as possible, taking his pension, and finding other work. Accordingly, that is recommended.

V

Hypochondriasis and Pain

One of the features common to chronic pain patients, both psychogenic and somatogenic, is hypochondriasis. This has been shown by psychological test results and the findings from clinical psychiatric interviews. With respect to test profiles, hypochondriacal items contribute substantially to neuroticism scores. For example, there are thirty-three Hypochondriasis (Hs) items in the Minnesota Multiphasic Personality Inventory, which essentially constitute a symptom checklist; twenty of these items also contribute to the sixty-item Hysteria scale. Thus, judgments about patients' neuroticism is, in part at least, greatly determined by their degree of hypochondriasis.

What is hypochondriasis? If a pain patient is hypochondriacal does it mean that his pain is "imaginary," or not real?

There have been many definitions of the term and there is little agreement about it. Without going into all of them we will adopt as most practical the definition put forward by Ladee (40): Hypochondriasis is a *"fascinated absorption by the experience of a physical or mental impairment."*

This definition has a number of advantages over others. "Fascinated absorption" conveys the sense of the patient's experience of being virtually helpless to change his preoccupation with his physical or mental condition, even as an obsessive neurotic may detest his ruminations but be unable to stop them. The "experience" is all important as this condition, like the experience of pain, is a subjective one whose existence must be inferred by an observer from what the patient says or does. "Physical or mental impairment" covers those patients who are afraid or convinced they are going crazy as well as those who are afraid or convinced they have a physical ailment.

Nowhere in this definition is there an objective standard of the patient's health, such as "complains of symptoms to a greater degree than is warranted by the facts." This is not a necessary condition, and in fact, it impairs the definition by presuming that if someone were to find an objective basis for the complaints, there would be no hypochondriasis. In fact, it is the "fascinated absorption with the experience of impairment" which constitutes the hypochondriasis, and this applies whether there are adequate objective mental or physical findings or not.

Thus the answer to the second question is, no, hypochondriasis does not mean that a pain (or any other symptom) is "imaginary," that requires a separate and independent determination. Patient A may have pain associated with an adequate organic lesion and yet go on living a satisfying life; he is not hypochondriacal. Patient B may have the same lesion and be almost totally preoccupied by it; he is hypochondriacal, inasmuch as the same mental mechanisms are involved in the production of hypochondriasis and psychogenic pain. It is quite rare, in my experience and that of other clinicians, to find a patient with psychogenic pain who is not absorbed by it to some degree.

Thus far, we have been speaking of hypochondriasis as though it were like pregnancy: one either has it or one doesn't. In fact, there is a spectrum of hypochondriasis just as there is of pain. For the latter, it ranges from twinges and aches that one hesitates to call pain, to the severest forms of tic douloureux which formerly drove many people to suicide. Similarly, there is a spectrum of concern about one's health, ranging from concern over diet, weight, and smoking, to an all-consuming delusion which most observers would agree is psychotic. The former we consider "normal" or "healthy," but there is a point at which it shades into something else that we think a bit neurotic, or at least eccentric, and that is usually when the other person is somewhat more preoccupied with, for example, his cholesterol intake than we are. We need now to understand more about the facts of hypochondriasis and the mechanisms involved.

THE STRUCTURE OF HYPOCHONDRIASIS

Scales like the MMPI Hs scale contain questions relating to each possible kind of symptom, such as "Do you often feel as if there were a tight band about your head?" and the number of such questions affirmatively answered is the measure of hypochondriasis. The effect of this is that a factor analysis results in such "factors" of hypochondriasis as "Bad Eyesight," "Poor Bowel Function," and "Sinusitis" (17), although Comrey was able to extract a major factor of Poor Physical Health (seventeen items) and a lesser one of Hypochondriasis (six items). He suggested that the chief factor would be better labeled Health Concern.

Pilowsky (58), however, began with definitions of hypochondriasis provided by 100 hospital staff members, and used elements of the most frequent statements to construct a twenty-item questionnaire. Items such as "Do you often worry about the possibility that you have got a serious illness?" show that this questionnaire is concerned primarily with patients' attitudes to disease and the reactions of others about them, rather than particular physical or mental symptoms.

Pilowsky showed that this questionnaire, which he named the "Whiteley Index," successfully discriminated between 100 psychiatric patients with hypochondriacal features and 100 psychiatric patients with few signs of hypochondriasis. The questionnaire also discriminated between the hypochondriacal patients and patients with cancer, and between the former and normal controls. (See also the study by Bond, ref. 8.) Evidence was presented of quite satisfactory test–retest reliability, and of validity as determined by correlations with scores from a questionnaire filled in by patients' relatives.

Of particular usefulness to our inquiry is the factor analysis performed by Pilowsky on the answers to the questionnaire. A factor analysis determines the patterns of responses to each of the items and identifies those which seem associated or clustered together. From this analysis, Pilowsky identified three factors, or elements which seem basic to the concept of hypochondriasis:

1. bodily preoccupation
2. disease phobia
3. conviction of the presence of disease with nonresponse to reassurance

Is it plain that these factors capture the flavor of the definition provided by Ladee (40) in that they seem clearly to represent a "fascinated absorption by the experience of a physical or mental impairment," and so, indirectly, the study by Pilowsky (58) lends support to the clinical and theoretical ideas in Ladee's definition. However, what is of interest is that the three factors are separate—by definition—in that factor analysis is concerned with identifying those items which are intercorrelated, and that the factors share little variance in common.

Thus, it is possible for a hypochondriacal patient to present with only one of the three elements, any combination of two, or perhaps all three. This would represent the spectrum from obsessive or phobic neurosis to psychotic (paranoid or depressive) delusion. It conforms to the idea of there existing a continuum of bodily concern ranging from healthy or normal to delusional.

A different sort of study altogether was performed by Kenyon (37), who examined the records of all patients seen at the Bethlem Royal and Maudsley Hospitals in the 10-year period from 1951–1960, and selected those receiving a solitary or primary diagnosis of hypochondriasis ($N = 301$) for comparison with those receiving a diagnosis of hypochondriasis secondary to some other diagnosis

($N = 211$). This is an epidemiological type of study; on some variables the groups were not only compared with each other, but with all patients seen in that period.

Of interest is that when diagnoses were compared in order to find the most frequently associated conditions, affective disorders and organic states were equally likely (11.6% each) to be the secondary diagnosis in the group with primary hypochondriasis (64.4% of whom received a diagnosis of hypochondriasis only). By comparison, of those receiving a secondary diagnosis of hypochondriasis, 82.4% received a primary diagnosis of an affective disorder.

From the histories of the current illness, the symptom most frequently presented was pain–occurring in 75% of the primary group and 62% of the secondary group. Affective symptoms, anxiety and depression, were next frequent, being present in about 40% of the primary group and 60% of the secondary group. Note how this supports the clinical and test findings of Pilling *et al.* (57) and the other studies cited earlier, that when pain is present it seems to mask anxiety or depression.

Kenyon also found that the most frequent complaints in both groups involved the head and neck, more than half the patients having symptoms referrable to this area, the abdomen and chest being the second and third sites involved. Findings made on inpatients (118 in the primary group and 177 in the secondary group) showed that 47.4% of each had no physical abnormalities, but that 44% of the former and 62.7% of the latter group showed signs of depression.

There were no significant differences between the groups with respect to age, sex, religion, social class, or marital status. They were also similar with respect to premobid personality, I.Q., physical disabilities, mental state, sexual adjustment, school and work history, past psychiatric history, family psychiatric history, and precipitating factors. The groups differed only in that those with a primary or exclusive diagnosis of hypochondriasis were likely to have had a longer history of the present illness with a less phasic course, fewer overt affective signs, were less likely to have received electroshock treatment, were less likely to be classed as recovered at discharge, and were more likely to receive a change in diagnosis at follow-up, this being to a psychiatric one.

Kenyon concludes that hypochondriasis is not a nosological entity, but a part of another syndrome, usually an affective one. From his data it would seem that a patient would, in lieu of experiencing depression, present himself to a hospital with a headache or stomachache.

Kreitman *et al.* (39) did a more intensive investigation of a small group of patients. They set up a hypochondriasis clinic in a general hospital, and selected 21 patients with depressive illness and marked somatic hypochondriacal syndromes. These were matched with 21 psychiatric patients with depressive illnesses with no somatic complaints. With this type of control they hoped to elucidate the processes of somatization.

They were not able to show that the hypochondriacal patients had a greater degree of social isolation, nor that they came from a lower socioeconomic class, or from families in which greater importance was placed on physical illness. They did find, however, that these patients were twice as likely as controls to have had a history of psychosomatic diseases before adulthood. The patients were also more likely than controls to have a poorer marital and sexual adjustment.

The somatizing patients, as compared with the nonsomatizing depressives, were more likely to have had the current illness precipitated by an external stress such as a death or illness, and also to have had a longer history of the present illness. Their symptoms were more like those of their mothers' (but not their fathers'). Interestingly, they had less depressive affect, although depressive mood was equally intense in both groups, and less evidence of anxiety, and the current illness caused less disruption of social, family, or occupational activities.

Once again we see evidence for the use of somatic symptoms as a defense against intolerable affect, and the suggestion that this pattern of response to stress was learned in childhood, perhaps with the mother as a model. In this connection, Walters (89) has observed that in his series of 430 patients with psychogenic regional pain, an association could usually be found among the site of the pain, a prior emotional hurt involving the same site, and a current situation evocative of the prior emotional hurt. Engel (23) and Szasz (82) have made similar observations.

This brings us then to the question of the psychodynamic mechanism involved in the production of hypochondriacal symptoms. The traditional psychoanalytic view is that it involves the withdrawal of cathexis, or libidinal energy, from external objects or relationships, which becomes displaced to the body in a form of narcissistic regression (16). In simpler terms, in the face of interpersonal pain or where needs are not being met, the patient regresses to a position in which he fusses over his health as he would have liked his mother to fuss over him when he was small.

We have seen that hypochondriacal complaints are associated with affective disorders, most often with depression, and this suggests not merely the additional association with chronicity, but a mechanism relating to the experience of loss and/or intropunitive anger. As in the production of psychogenic pain, which may be only one of a number of hypochondriacal complaints, the patient may have experienced a real or imaginary loss of someone close to him, or similarly some loss or decline of body function or skill, or be similarly disappointed with respect to his job or career.

It is striking that the mean age of the patients in almost all the studies cited is about 42 years. In our Western culture this is the time when one is well into middle age, when children are maturing and husband and wife are again the center of each other's attention, and when one has usually reached the limits of occupational success. In all of these areas there are bases for disappointment and discouragement. Middle age is also the time when anxiety-provoking stresses occur. Friends die of heart attacks. One reads of famous persons, younger than oneself, being treated for cancer. Parents die, and one wonders whether (and when) one will die of the same disease. With the advancing years there is a clearly noticeable increase in uncomfortable physical sensations; joints ache, muscles stiffen, more foods are harder to digest, and sleep comes less easily and is less restful.

With such mundane sources of concern, the ground is laid for a hypochondriacal reaction. A typical sequence is essentially as follows: there are difficulties at home or at work, consisting primarily of a failure to receive recognition or other needs, and this results in feelings of resentment and self-pity, which cannot be expressed appropriately. There are physical changes consisting of increased numbers of new and uncomfortable feelings, in a setting of increased concerns about health in friends and relatives. Suddenly the individual is not merely noticing physical sensations but he is becoming worried about them, and he finds himself half convinced that he has a certain serious disease. Feelings of dread well up within him and soon he finds himself making appointments with doctors.

Such a pattern of events is supported by reports in the clinical literature and also by the objective studies we have cited. The question may arise, "Why doesn't everybody become a hypochondriac under such conditions?" Clearly, not everyone develops stress-response symptoms. Among those who do, some develop other psychiatric illnesses; some "act out" by becoming alcoholic or quitting their homes or jobs; and some develop physical disorders. Those who become hypochondriacal seem to have been prepared for this in childhood by having reacted to stresses with psychophysiological disorders, perhaps resulting in favorable attention from an otherwise cold and controlling mother (40), with whose physical symptoms the patient identified (39). With respect to premobid personality, there is little consistency—both hysterical and obsessive–compulsive personalities being common—although Ladee (40) feels that virtually all such patients are outwardly assertive yet inwardly very unsure of themselves, and have an excessive dependency on one of the parents (or parent–surrogate), usually the mother.

CASE ILLUSTRATION 3

Mr. C. Mc. is a 56-year-old retired Navy officer who is admitted for evaluation of intractable low-back pain of 3-year duration, and is referred by a private orthopedist.

Relevant History. Mr. Mc.'s difficulties began about 2 months after retirement, when he lifted a heavy object and experienced sudden pain down his left leg. Conservative treatment failed, and despite negative myelograms, neurosurgical judgment indicated that intervention was indicated, and consequently, the patient had a disc excised. The patient was told that severe arachnoiditis was noted. Since surgery, the radicular pain disappeared, but severe low-back pain radiating from the site of the laminectomy has persisted, with relief only obtained from medication.

There is a significant drug problem, in that the patient originally took three Percodan per day, but now takes one Percodan, two Empirim #3, and 8–10 oz. of bourbon per day, to kill the pain.

There is no compensation issue. Mr. Mc. gets about $12,000 yearly retirement, plus about $3000 from Social Security. He has no friends in this area, and sees only his immediate family, and apparently, doctors whom he visits regularly. He likes to play golf, but says he cannot at present.

Test Findings. Mr. Mc. endorsed a highly significant number of items on the Health Index in all four areas: chronic invalidism, manifest depression, pain preoccupation, and playing pain games with doctors. This is a neurotic pattern.

He estimates the intensity of his usual pain as 50 on a 0–100 scale, a moderate amount. However, on the tourniquet ischemic pain test, his usual clinical pain was matched after only 4 sec, while his maximum tolerance was reached in 5 min 20 sec, making his usual clinical pain only 1% of tolerance, or a trivial amount. (His very worst exacerbated pain was matched at 2 min 30 sec, or at 47% of tolerance.) This difference between his pain estimation of 50 and pain matching of 1% suggests that his perception and/or reporting are distorted, perhaps by a neurotic problem.

The MMPI profile shows a highly significant neurotic pattern, with a clear tendency to somatic complaints and strong features of hypochondriasis and anxiety (Fig. 10). There is also a slight amount of depression. The pattern is less

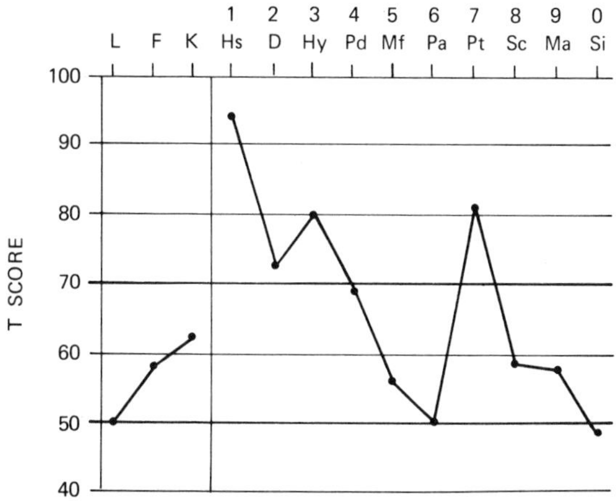

Fig. 10. MMPI profile of patient C. Mc.

that of the usual psychophysiological disorder, masking depression and anxiety, but more that of an anxiety neurosis with somatic features.

Diagnostic Impression. Anxiety neurosis, moderate (330.07), with hypochondriasis.

Recommendations. It would seem that Mr. Mc. has focused on his injured back a number of his intrapsychic and interpersonal problems, only a few of which are obvious. In discussing these findings with him, he readily agreed to them, and admitted to having a Physicians' Desk Reference and Merck Manual in which he read extensively. It was pointed out that his payoffs for having pain included the justifying of his excessive drug and alcohol intake (considering the very slight amount of pain), and not having to make friends. He agreed to come off narcotics entirely, and as liver function tests were normal (given his drinking history, this needed to be checked), he was prescribed amitriptyline, 75 mg q.h.s., and diazepam 10 mg and acetaminophen 650 mg q.4.h. while awake. Psychiatric referral was recommended, but the patient declined.

ABNORMAL ILLNESS BEHAVIOR

Pilowsky (60) notes that the fuzzy definitions of hysteria, functional overlay, hypochondriasis, somatization reactions, etc., have led to inappropriate diagnoses and uncertain management of patients who complain of physical symptoms in the absence of an adequate organic cause. He proposes that instead of the traditional sick-role concept, which influences both the illness behavior of the patient and the reactions of others about him, a concept of "illness behavior" should be adopted.

Illness behavior refers to the "ways in which symptoms may be differentially perceived, evaluated, and acted (or not acted) upon by different kinds of persons (45)." Pilowsky suggests that if the doctor does not believe that the patient's objective pathology is significant, and if the patient's illness behavior is uninfluenced by the doctor's explanations, then the patient may be said to show "abnormal illness behavior."

The emphasis here is on the patient's response to the doctor's explanation and recommendations (based upon thorough examination). If the patient accepts the doctor's findings and recommendations, there is no abnormal illness behavior; if he does not, there is. Abnormal illness behavior, therefore, can apply as a concept no matter what psychiatric diagnosis, if any, is made (61). Focusing upon the patient's reaction to explanation and prescription in this fashion has the advantage of bringing in certain concepts from medical sociology and social psychology. Mechanic (46), for example, uses attribution theory to describe the ways in which persons respond to perceptions of body sensations with illness behavior. The usual initial hypochondriacal complaint is nonspecific and similar to frequently occurring symptoms in the normal population, as symptoms of responses to stress. The diffuseness and commonness are conditions under which very many attributions (causal explanations) may occur. When ordinary symptoms occur with emotional arousal, and are not easily explained in conventional and commonly understood ways, the individual casts about for external cues to define the meaning and importance of the symptoms.

Sociocultural factors determine whether an individual will use the vocabulary of emotional or of bodily complaints when seeking relief from stressful situations. Orientations due to ethnic membership influence help-seeking behavior (95), and indeed it has been shown that such cultural differences influence not merely the perception of pain but the physiological responses to painful stimuli (78,87). Many patients express psychological distress through a physical language, not merely because the concept of psychological distress has not been taught them but the very vocabulary for such a concept is lacking. Thus Merskey and Spear (53) note that it took many months of intensive psychotherapy for a patient to quit complaining of pain and instead to talk about her intolerable "tension" (p. 75).

Unfortunately, few studies in the sociological field concerning pain and hypochondriasis meet current criteria of methodological rigor, and our information in this area is still incomplete (92). The review of Mechanic (46) nonetheless suggests that we may add another dimension to the purely psychodynamic model of hypochondriasis presented earlier. That is, the somatization process may be described in terms of withdrawal of cathexis from external objects; or it may be described in terms of a learned use of physical illness as a mode of expressing and resolving conflicts.

In light of this, Pilowsky (61) suggests that abnormal illness behavior be diagnosed by concurrent mental status and physical examinations, including consideration of current sources of emotional conflicts and background sociocultural factors. In other words, traditional hypochondriasis should be diagnosed not merely by ruling out organic factors, or excluding physical causes as an adequate explanation, but by making positive psychosocial findings as well. This is particularly important when evaluating the hypochondriasis of the somatogenic pain patient. Here the issue is more clearly not one of "imaginary" versus "real," but one of the "fascinated absorption" which prevents the patient from leading a satisfying life despite his pain. Inasmuch as there are pain patients who can surmount their pain, we must look to the psychological and social variables for understanding and treating the patient who cannot.

VI

Pain and Depression

Most psychiatric texts and references do not mention pain in connection with depression, even though pain complaints appear in their case illustrations. As an example of how pain can be omitted from a list of depressive symptoms, Zung's (96) Self-Rating Depression scale is composed of twenty items collated from several published descriptions of the syndrome, but contains no item concerning pain. Similarly, the Depression scale of the well-known and much-used Minnesota Multiphasic Personality Inventory contains sixty items, including nine which overlap with the Hypochondriasis scale, but none of the sixty has pain in the content. Yet clinical interpretation of an elevated Depression score, especially in conjunction with elevations on the Hysteria or Hypochondriasis scales, almost routinely predicts pain complaints.

This leads then to the question of incidence: How common is pain in depression? A few studies have reported on pain symptoms in depressed patients, although with quite variable results according to the rigor with which the study was done. For example, Diamond (21) reported that of 423 patients with various types of depression, 84% had headaches as one of their complaints or only complaint. Diagnosis was made on the basis of disturbances of sleep, weight, and libido.

In a similarly uncontrolled study, Lesse (42) reported that of 324 depressed patients seen by him 31% had masked depressions, that is, major presenting symptoms related to various organ systems, some of which undoubtedly involved pain complaints.

In contrast, Cassidy *et al.* (14) made a careful study of the symptoms and signs in 100 severely depressed manic depressives, as compared with several control groups. Pain was not used as a diagnostic criterion, but was solicited

TABLE 6.1 Percentage of Groups Acknowledging Pain Symptoms[a]

Type of pain	Manic-depressives $N = 100$ (94 depressed)	Anxiety neurotics $N = 134$	Female hysterics $N = 50$	Medically sick controls $N = 50$	Healthy controls $N = 246$
Headache	49	65	94	36	25
Chest	36	81		50	8
Abdominal	38		78	38	16
Back	39		56	40	16
Joint	30		28	22	5
Extremity	25		62	26	5

[a] Adapted from data in Cassidy *et al.* (14), by permission of W. L. Cassidy and the *Journal of the American Medical Association.*

from patients by interview and checklist, along with other symptoms. If we abstract pain symptoms from the others, and combine results from several of their tables, we can summarize their findings in Table 6.1.

The significance of differences among the groups is not apparent, and we do not have an idea of the variability from this table. But it seems apparent that the complaint of pain is a sign of illness, although it is about as equally likely to be a sign of psychiatric illness as of physical illness. Pain is not associated with depression more than other psychiatric classifications, but is present more often than in healthy controls, even as it is present more in physical disease than in health. This point was stated quite clearly also by Stengel (69).

Watts (90) wrote of the "mild endogenous depressions" which rarely are seen by psychiatrists and seem to be a type of disease seen by general practitioners. In describing the presenting symptom in 100 cases, there were 6 with headache, 4 with chest pain, 3 with back pain, and 2 with muscular pains, for a total of 15% with pain as the chief complaint. Watts felt that the mild endogenous depression could appear frankly as an overt depression, or masquerade as another psychiatric disturbance such as an anxiety state, or as a "depressive equivalent" simulating an organic illness, or as a "depressive graft," grafted onto an organic illness.

In addition to looking at the incidence of pain in depression, we may consider the incidence of depression (and other diagnoses) in patients with pain complaints. The work of Merskey and Separ (53) reviews their own and others' studies. In one of their studies they found that in 200 consecutive admissions to a psychiatric clinic, pain was a symptom in 106 (53%). Depression was the most common diagnosis, 85 of 200, and pain occurred in 48 of the 85 depressive (56%). The next most common diagnosis was anxiety hysteria, and pain was a symptom in 40 of 76 of these patients (53%). In a comparable study in a general medical practice, Baker and Merskey (3) found that 176 of 276 consecutive patients (64%) had pain, and 78 of the 276 were thought to have primarily a psychiatric disorder. Of the 198 "organics," 66% had pain complaints, and of the 78 "psychiatric" patients, 59% had pain complaints.

In the report by Pilling *et al.* (57) referred to previously, 562 patients were seen in psychiatric consultation. Of these, 32% had pain as a *presenting* complaint, and depression was found to be significantly less frequent in both men and women with pain than those without pain. Of 221 men, 41 of 65 (63%) with pain were thought to have depressive symptoms, while 120 of 156 (77%) without pain had these symptoms. There were comparable differences among the 341 women: of the 117 with pain, 76 (65%) were depressed, while of the 224 without pain, 177 (79%) were depressed.

It appears, then, that the complaint of pain occurs in slightly more than half the general medical and psychiatric populations, and in psychiatric populations the presence of a pain complaint is about equally likely to predict a diagnosis of anxiety hysteria or reactive depression. There is a tendency for pain, like other somatic complaints, to "mask" depression, so that patients with pain complaints are somewhat less likely to receive a diagnosis of depression than are those who do not have such complaints of pain.

Another way of studying the relationship of pain and depression is to see what happens to the pain complaint when the depression is relieved. Bradley (12) studied the response to antidepressant treatment of two groups of patients: 16 whose pain preceded the depression, and 19 whose pain and depression occurred together. In the first group, depression alone responded to treatment, but there was an increased tolerance to the pain. In the second group, both the pain and the depression were relieved by treatment of the depression.

Having established that there is a relationship between pain and depression, we need to examine in some greater detail what constitutes depression.

THE ELEMENTS OF DEPRESSION

The items used in the Minnesota Multiphasic Personality Inventory were empirically derived on the basis of their ability to discriminate among diagnostic groups. On the basis of subjective item analysis, Harris and Lingoes (32) grouped the sixty items on the Depression scale into five subscales which seem to reflect the components of depression. These components are

1. *subjective depression,* joylessness, pessimism, low self-esteem
2. *psychomotor retardation,* nonparticipation in social relations
3. Complaints about *physical malfunctioning,* self-preoccupation
4. *Mental dullness* and unresponsiveness
5. *Brooding,* ruminativeness, irritability

This is a listing of the characteristics common to the items which seemed correlated, on a subjective basis. A more rigorous search for the components of depression would require a factor analysis. Meanwhile, before examining such studies, it is well to note that subscale 3 is of interest to us in that it consists of items related to physical malfunctioning to which patients usually assume pain refers.

Comrey (18) used a sample of 360 subjects, including 85 Veterans Administration psychiatric patients of various diagnoses, and 80 college students who had applied for personal counseling, and performed a factor analysis of the MMPI Depression scale items. He obtained nine factors which he could label, but most of these were trivial and had only a few items in them. The main factor was *Neuroticism,* and contained twenty-six of sixty items on the scale, and Comrey suggested that the scale be relabeled Neuroticism and include just those twenty-six items. Two other factors of interest emerged, one called *Poor Physical Health,* consisting of thirteen items related to health concerns and similar to Harris and Lingoes' subscale of physical malfunctioning; and the other called *Depression,* consisting of five items of manifest depression, which is similar to Harris and Lingoes' subscale of subjective depression.

These two analyses of one particular scale seem to suggest that depression consists of several components at least: subjective feelings of depression; overconcern with physical health; and some general complaining, neurotic, or irritability factor. To determine the generality of these, we will have to consider several studies which use other tests or scales, and see what emerges.

Hamilton (31) examined 49 depressed male patients, and used seventeen variables including personality traits, symptoms, and signs. As a result of his analysis, four factors emerged, two of which seemed particularly clear. One was a factor of *Retarded Depression,* and another was a factor of *Agitation and Somatic Symptoms.* The other factors seemed related to an anxiety reaction, and to insomnia and somatic symptoms, but these were weaker factors.

Overall (54) used thirty-one rating measures on 204 hospitalized depressive patients. He extracted seven factors.

1. *Depression in mood*
2. *Guilt*
3. *Anxiety*
4. *Psychomotor retardation*
5. *Subjective experience of illness*
6. *Abnormal preoccupation with physical health*
7. *Physiological reaction to stress*

If factors 1, 2, and 5 are combined, we are again left with subjective depression, hypochondriasis, retardation, and somatic symptoms, and an anxiety or agitation factor.

Friedman *et al.* (27) studied 170 psychotic depressed patients, using a sixty-item list of traits, symptoms, and themes, twenty-two of which were factor analyzed. The result yielded four psychotic depressive syndromes, or types:

1. *Classical mood or affective depression,* including feelings of guilt, loss of self-esteem, doubt, and psychological internalizing tendencies
2. *Retardation,* a withdrawn and apathetic depression
3. *"Biological" reactions,* with loss of appetite, sleep disturbance, constipation, work inhibition, and loss of satisfaction
4. *Hypochondriacal type,* querulous, self-preoccupied, demanding and complaining, irritable, with marked body consciousness, and many physical complaints. This was not the "somatic equivalent" of depression, as these patients ate and slept better than the "biological" types.

This last syndrome or "type" is a little different from the factors previously reported, in that it combines the elements of irritability and complaining with that of bodily preoccupation; however, it does support the previous findings of an important hypochondriacal element in depression, along with the retardation, somatic symptoms, and subjective depression. The main psychological theme for these hypochondriacal depressive types, according to Friedman *et al.,* is oral frustration; these patients being clinging and demanding and quite threatened by separation anxiety.

Thus far we have considered studies which either examined psychotic depressives alone, or looked at depression in all psychiatric and normal subjects. However, it is well known that "depression" may refer to an entire spectrum of feelings and behaviors, ranging from discouragement and dejection in normals to say, involutional psychotic depression. If factor analysis is to discriminate among the components of depression, it should be sensitive to these differences which may not merely be differences in degree, but differences in kind. For our purposes, we are particularly interested in what may be called the neurotic or reactive depressives, inasmuch as this seems to be the single most common diagnosis or characteristic of chronic-pain patients.

One of the early and classical reports on the likelihood of there being two different kinds of depression, endogenous and reactive, was that of Kiloh and Garside (38). These authors studied 143 patients, 53 with endogenous depression and 90 with neurotic depression, using thirty-five items consisting of personality traits and characteristics of the present illness. Two factors were obtained from their analysis, the second one accounting for most of the variance and being clearly associated with the two types of depression. That is, many of the items discriminated very well between the two types, being positive for one and negative for the other, showing a clear difference between endogenous and reactive depression.

Kay *et al.* (35) extended this finding of the two kinds of depression, using a thirty-five item scale consisting of psychiatric and physical findings, precipitants, social and personality features, and other items. Their subjects were 104 patients drawn equally from a general hospital and a mental hospital, made up of 35 with endogenous depression, 27 with involutional depression, 27 with neurotic depression, and 15 with paranoid states. Their first factor, accounting for most of the variance, seemed to be bipolar; at one end were clustered guilt, retardation, severe depression, hopelessness, suicidal behavior, ideas of nihilism and reference, and hallucinations; at the other end were somatic complaints, blaming others, early wakening and worse mood in the morning, initial insomnia, and weight loss. Thus one pole seemed to be associated with endogenous retarded depressions, and these patients were described as having narrow interests and tended to be treated with electroconvulsive therapy. The other pole was associated with neurotic complaining depression, and these patients were described as having psychogenic disorders with their illnesses tending to have persisted longer than 1 year. Kay *et al.* also found a second, weaker factor which seemed to separate depressives and paranoids, but this is of lesser interest to our inquiry, although we shall return to it when we consider the dynamics of depression.

Pilowsky *et al.* (63) also examined the question of whether depression consists of two separate types, but rather than using factor analysis they employed regular statistical analyses of items and compared groups on these. They administered a fifty-seven-item scale to 200 mental patients, including 38 with endogenous depression and 38 with reactive depression. On the bases of item analyses, they came up with three groups.

Class A: A mixed group of depressive reactions, whose characteristics included daytime depression worsening in the evening, environmental problems, bodily concerns, and loss of interests.

Class B: The endogenous depressions, characterized by depression, retardation, and loss of interests, appetite, sleep, libido, and ability to concentrate.

Class C: The nondepressive illness.

These groupings support the previous findings of differences between the neurotic and endogenous depressions, and seem also to support the idea that hypochondriasis seems to be associated with the neurotic depression which is reactive to environmental precipitants.

Finally, Kear-Colwell (36) examined 203 mental patients of whom 102 were depressed, including 49 with endogenous depression and 42 with reactive depression. He used a list of fifty-four items containing depressive phenomena and antecedent events. Six relevant factors were extracted:

1. Loss of appetite, tiredness, difficulty in concentration, loss of interests, lack of pleasure.
2. Guilt, self-deprecation, agitation.
3. Bereavement, loss of weight, concern about physical health.

4. Retardation, family history of depression, denial of feelings of alienation.
5. Sleep disturbance, environmental precipitants, derealization.
6. Suicidal ideation, unhappy thoughts.

All the factors except Factor 4 differentiated between depressives and others. Factors 4 and 5 discriminated between the endogenous and the reactive depressions: Factor 4 was positive for the endogenous patients, negative for the reactive patients; Factor 5 was positive for the reactive patients, negative for the endogenous patients. If we consider that bereavement is a response to an environmental precipitant (Factor 3), then hypochondriasis again is seen to be associated with neurotic depressive reactions, although in this study it failed to discriminate between the two groups of depressives.

In general, these studies show that there are two main forms of depression. Endogenous or psychotic depression appears to be characterized by retardation or agitation, guilt, somatic disturbances, early morning awakening, and morning accentuation of mood; it is associated with a family history of depression. Reactive or neurotic depression seems to be characterized by tiredness, loss of interests, hypochondriacal complaints, daytime depression with evening accentuation of mood; it is a persistent response to an environmental precipitant.

Findings such as these support the earlier suggestions from the literature on psychogenic pain patients that the pain seems to be a particular kind of bodily preoccupation taken as a response to some external stress. The neurotic depression too can be seen as a natural response of those with organic pain generators to the persistent pain and disability. Anxious complaining and depressive mood are characteristic of both kinds of chronic pain patients, and it seems as though it makes little difference whether the precipitant is an environmental or an organic one, the outcome seems so similar.

This is not to suggest that all pain patients receive a diagnosis of neurotic depression, for certainly they do not, and, as we have seen, anxiety hysteria is almost as common in the psychogenic pain group. But it is the most common diagnosis, and in the organic pain group, it seems to be the most common pattern in those whose pain has been moderate to severe and persistent. Pain complaints are also seen in patients with schizophrenic and endogenous depression, but much less frequently so than in the neurotic disorders.

In particular, it is important to note that the somatic disorders which accompany endogenous depression, and sometimes mask it, are different from (and appear in different factors than) the bodily preoccupation and somatic complaints of the neurotic depression. The former seems attributable to the neurochemical changes which have been found in the psychotic depressions, and the latter, the hypochondriasis, seems associated with the interpersonal coping style in the reactive disorder.

CASE ILLUSTRATION 4

Mrs. G. M. is a 70-year old widow referred by a private physician because of pain "in the tailbone," which came on following a hard bump while horseback riding 10 years ago. Neurological examination is entirely normal.

Relevant History. Following the accident Mrs. M. received a number of therapies, including medications and cortisone injections, and 6 years ago had an excision of the coccyx. This resulted in continued pain which she says is now worse than it was preoperatively. Other than the change in intensity, the pain has retained the same quality for 10 years: it is a severe "bone" pain which has a boring, "bruiselike" quality which is present constantly, is made worse by sitting, "hurts terribly when I lay down," usually awakens her from sleep about 3:00 AM, and allows her to fall asleep only by taking sleeping tablets and meprobamate. There are no bowel or bladder dysfunctions, no weakness or pain in the legs, and there is no change in pain with the usual things that make low-back pain worse.

Mrs. M. is a big-boned, active woman who looks more like a 50 year old than a 70 year old; she seems to need activity. She grew up in the West. Her father was a minister who had a family history of tuberculosis and so moved to the desert climate, however he was unaware that he had heart trouble and died of a heart attack aggravated by the high altitude when he was 46. He also had an accident prior to marriage and had epilepsy, with seizures occurring about every 6 months.

The patient's mother was a housewife who lived to be 88. The patient has two younger sisters, and a brother who died about 4 years ago with Parkinson's disease.

After the patient finished school in the West, she went East to continue her schooling for a year, then returned to take a clerical job, which she has held off and on until about 8 years ago. At 21 she had married a cattleman. He was a disabled World War I veteran who, like her father, had tuberculosis and a bad heart, and after 46 years of marriage he died.

Mrs. M. had three children: a daughter who died at 9 from typhoid fever brought into the home by a carrier; a son who is now 44 and teaches art in a nearby high school; and a son who is now 29 and lives with her—he is mentally retarded, has cerebral palsy, and epilepsy. She is quite concerned about his future; although her other son will provide for him after she dies, she worries about his social life—she now takes him to various social events for retarded persons.

Mrs. M. lives on Social Security and an annuity from the Federal Retirement fund including a supplement for her son. She takes no prescription analgesics. Some days she takes two aspirins 2–3 times a day, other days she takes none, as they upset her stomach. She takes the sleeping medication and two meprobamate at night, and 25 mg of amitriptyline each morning.

Test Findings. On the Health Index, Mrs. M. endorsed a significant number of items relating to chronic invalidism, manifest depression, almost all the items concerning problems with doctors, but only a moderate number relating to pain preoccupation. The pattern suggests that psychological problems may be making a significant contribution to her pain.

Mrs. M. estimates the usual severity of her pain as 50 on a scale of 0 to 100, a moderate amount. On the tourniquet pain test her clinical pain level was reached in 9 min 32 sec, and her maximum tolerance at 11 min 59 sec. This is a relatively high tolerance for women in our sample, and her clinical pain level is 80% of it, which indicates severe pain. Her estimate of 50 is considerably below this severe level, and along with her only moderate preoccupation with pain, it suggests that she is a noncomplainer.

Lack of complaining is often associated with introversion, and is also a part of her upbringing and ethnic background. Mrs. M.'s MMPI (Fig. 11) shows a high degree of introversion. In addition, her profile indicates a clinically significant reactive depression and some anxiety, accompanied by feelings of inadequacy and inefficiency. The depression is probably in part reactive to her physical symptoms and related difficulties in continuing to function well, but in turn it is undoubtedly potentiating her pain.

Diagnostic Impression. Depressive neurosis, mild (300.46), with anxiety.

Discussion and Recommendations. Mrs. M. has severe pain, more than she shows or lets on. Inasmuch as further surgical treatment is unlikely, the

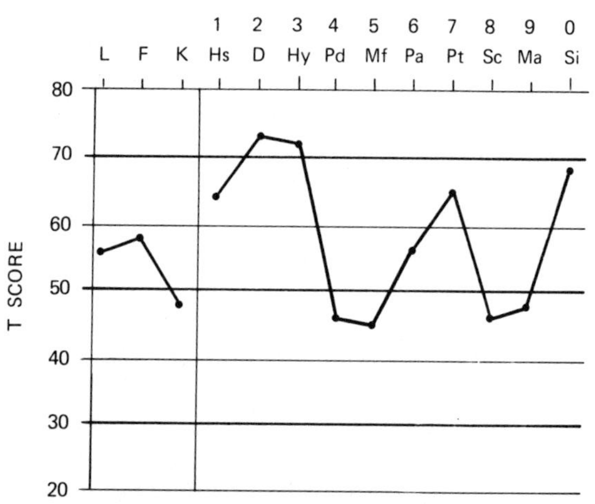

Fig. 11. MMPI profile of patient G. M.

psychological approach is most important. It is almost certain that her psychological state is contributing to the severity of her pain, but it must be kept in mind that the patient learned early in life, and frequently thereafter, that suffering was her lot in life, and bearing a cross is not at all foreign to her. Thus, with any significant reduction in pain, Mrs. M. would probably manage quite well.

It is unlikely that Mrs. M. needs inpatient rehabilitation; she is too active, and needs to keep moving. She would also worry too much about her youngest son to benefit from inpatient treatment. Accordingly, she should be managed by medications, as an outpatient. Her medications should be changed to: amitriptyline, 100 mg q.h.s; after 2 weeks, if there is no decreased pain, acetaminophen with codeine, $\frac{1}{4}$ gr., q.6.h while awake.

Follow-up. With the amitriptyline alone, Mrs. M. reported that her pain disappeared, and she slept well, after 2 weeks. A month later, she requested discontinuing the antidepressant as it made her too relaxed. She did so, and 2 weeks later called to say that her pain had returned as before. She was instructed to resume the previous dosage of amitriptyline, to which she agreed, preferring the relaxed feeling to the pain. Two weeks later she reported the pain had gone again.

THE DYNAMICS OF NEUROTIC DEPRESSION

We have already described the elements of reactive depression as the response to loss or intropunitive anger, and that the precipitants are likely to be events occurring at home or at work, the two areas in which people become emotionally involved. The loss may be an actual separation by death or departure, or an effective one such as withdrawal of affection or emotional estrangement. The anger may be an inexpressible one which is a reaction to a frustration, or to a real or imagined slight or insult; Bender's (5) case histories illustrate the role of suppressed anger in the production of somatic complaints.

We have also seen that there appears to be a bipolar representation of paranoid and depressive characteristics (35). The depressive position can be clarified by contrasting it with the paranoid position, in response to a loss, an insult, or an experience of pain.

Paranoid	*Depressive*
1. There is a cause	1. There is a cause
2. Outside forces are responsible	2. I am responsible
3. I must do something	3. Nothing can be done

The position of the paranoid patient results in abrasive behavior which irritates others, alienating them and confirming his views. The position of the depressive patient results in an expression of hopelessness which sucks others to him, to no avail, thus confirming his views.

The traditional psychodynamic view of depression is that it results from too severe a superego, the internalized reproving parent punishing the patient for unacceptable impulses of a sexual, dependent, or aggressive nature. Indeed, when hallucinations are present in the psychotic depressions, they are usually auditory and accusative; often the patient can identify the voice as belonging to one of his parents, and the accusation concerns some sinful behavior of the past, or one in which the patient might want to engage.

A modern psychodynamic view emphasizes the interpersonal approach to neurotic depression, which is appropriate since it is a response to an interpersonal event. In particular, Bonime (11) has described the *practice* of depression, stressing the powerfulness of the depressive position as an expression of a basically competitive personality. Depression is a practice which consists of manipulating others by expressions of dependency. Depression is further characterized by an aversion to influence by others, almost directly proportional to the patients' manipulativeness of others, and by an unwillingness to give gratification to others. It is a form of expressing anger, and thus hostility seems to be sensed by others who cannot quite pinpoint the reasons. The depressive attempts to get support and concern from others without incurring the responsibility for reciprocating. Although Bonime notes that all of this may lie outside the patient's awareness, the practice of depression may be observed in the nature of the interactions he has and the emotional reactions of others.

It should be obvious that the complaint of pain functions in much the same way as the expression of hopelessness, and we will consider the interpersonal aspects of pain in the next chapter. First, however, we should consider the physiological relationships of pain and depression.

PSYCHOPHYSIOLOGICAL MECHANISMS

The repeated association, in the studies cited, of chronic pain and depression has led some authors to speculate that one causes the other. It is, however, possible that both states may be caused by an independent third process. More exactly, we should say that when described psychologically, chronic pain and depression seem almost to be interchangeable: chronic pain usually leads to a reactive depression, and a reactive depression frequently results in complaints of pain.

This leads us then to hypothesize that, if these phenomena were to be described in physiological terms, certain mechanisms in common would be found. Unfortunately the research in this area is sparse. Most of the biochemical studies of depression in man have dealt with psychotic or endogenous depressive states, and there are virtually no studies of chronic pain states in which central neurochemical processes are measured. Nevertheless, there are some scattered preliminary reports which are suggestive.

A number of authors have noted that the tricyclic antidepressants, alone or in combination with phenothiazines, are effective in reducing or eliminating pain consequent to organic lesions (52). The tricyclic compounds are thought to have their effect by virtue of inhibiting the reuptake of norepinephrine by adrenergic neurons (34). This results in an increased sensitization to the catecholamine.

Recent studies by Akil (1) and Akil and Mayer (2) indicate that there is a monaminergically mediated pain inhibitory mechanism located in the mesencephalic ventral central gray area. Electrical stimulation of this area reliably produced analgesia in rats (44), and preliminary studies have indicated similar findings in cats (43). Augmentation of serotonin by injection of its precursor (5-HTP) augments the analgesia (1). Norepinephrine inhibits analgesia, while dopamine facilitates it, although the dopaminergic effect is dominant over that of norepinephrine (1). Battista and Wolff could alter the pain tolerance of patients by the administration of levodopa (4).

These findings, although quite preliminary, suggest that the relationship of pain and depression may lie in the balance of the brain monoamines. Low levels of the catecholamines are presumed to underly the depressions, and the effect of tricyclics and monoamine oxidase inhibitors in relieving depressions is presumed to lie in their ability to prevent degradation of the monamines. However, this is a nonspecific effect, and presumably both serotonin and norepinephrine levels are enhanced.

From the work of Akil (1) we may hypothesize that, at least in the mesencephalic central gray, norepinephrine diminishes the analgesic-mediating properties of serotonin and dopamine, and in this possibility may lie the reason why antidepressants are not always effective in controlling pain. One may speculate therefore that an agent which stimulates serotonin and/or dopamine activity without also raising norepinephrine levels, may be a more effective agent in relieving pain and the related depression.

This field, at any rate, seems to hold the promise for establishing the psychophysiological mechanisms shared by pain and depression, as these phenomena seem so often to be related in psychological terms.

VII

Pain Transactions

We have so far reviewed the major, most common features of patients with chronic pain, both with respect to objective psychological characteristics, and the presumed underlying psychodynamic mechanisms. This is a necessary prelude to a consideration of diagnosis and treatment, but it is incomplete without a review of the interpersonal aspects of pain. The interpersonal description of pain is less well known and understood than the more traditional approaches.

In a previous chapter we mentioned that Szasz (82) identified three levels of meaning of pain: the first as a subjective symptom; the second as a form of interpersonal behavior, requesting aid; and the third as a symbolic level, in which the pain represents some 'pain" in the individual's life and his method of coping with it. Engel (23) approached a similar analysis in distinguishing between the "peripheral signature" and the "individual psychic signature" of the description of pain, as aids in determining the psychogenic component of the pain. Szasz (83) explicitly detailed the use of pain as a symbol of interpersonal communication: as a request for help; as a statement that help is not possible; and as a symbolic warning of intrapsychic or interpersonal threat. In his paper Szasz takes the position that it is not always possible to translate the symbol "pain" into an interpretation of psychological distress which can then be resolved—sometimes there is no solution to the problem.

Later Szasz (84) expanded on this thesis, coining the term "painmanship" to describe the interaction which occurs between pain patients and doctors. In the game of painmanship, the physician's aim is to confirm his professional identity by being able to identify the cause of the pain, and to relieve the patient's suffering. The patient's aim, on the other hand, is to confirm his identity as a painful, suffering person by presenting with undiagnosable pain and unrelievable suffering. Szasz contends that it is as unreasonable to expect the patient to give up his identity and career, as it is to ask the physician to do so.

There are two problems here. One is that Szasz is talking about psychogenic pain patients primarily; the other is that the pain patient will not let doctors be: he insists on medical and surgical intervention which confirms his being a suffering person and legitimizes his role as a professional invalid. In addition, the patient ostensibly insists on relief, and it is very difficult for the doctor to differentiate between the patient who really wants relief, and the patient who demands it but does not intend to get well.

Berne (6) described some of the specific kinds of games patients play which are applicable to pain patients: "Veteran" ("I got my rights"), "Wooden Leg" ("What do you expect of a man with a wooden leg?"), and "Peasant" ["Thank you, Doctor, (but I'm no better)"]. An important point made by Berne, and the basic position put forth by Szasz, is that they are not describing "secondary gains" as this term is used in the traditional sense. The concept of "secondary gains" is valid only within the psychoanalytic model which assumes that masochism, or the experience of pain *per se*, is the "primary gain." This may be true of some pain patients, but the assumption must be validated in each case. For many pain patients, compensation, addiction, the confounding of doctors, or the sick role may be the major motivating factor.

DEFINITIONS AND WARNING

As we are using the term, following the work of Berne (6), a "game" is a series of transactions between two or more persons with an ulterior motive (communication on more than one level of meaning) and a payoff at the end of the series; it is a set of moves with a "gimmick" at the end. A game in this sense is not a pastime engaged in for fun. There is no assumption that the patient (or doctor) is aware of what he is doing, or that the motives are conscious; this is unnecessary in describing the moves which are actually made.

A "life-style" is a series of games over a period of time designed to confirm and display a particular self-concept. Some persons engage in a variety of games to show they are alcoholics, drug addicts, doctors, or pain patients. A life-style includes professional career and reflection of the self. It is the outward answer to the question, "What are you?" Berne (7) refers to persons' "scripts," by which he means a life plan decided on in childhood, partially programmed by parents, and partly determined by life events; it is analogous to the "repetition compulsion" of psychoanalytic theory. We prefer to use the term "life-style" because it implies less about causative factors, and better takes into account the purely fortuitous life event (accident or illness) which can markedly alter a person's way of living.

The approach to be described here is sometimes accused of being cynical, just as psychoanalysis was once accused of being "dirty" because it uncovered hidden sexual bases of behavior. Viewing the games played by doctors and patients may seem cynical because it focuses on their actual behavior, and ignores the purity of motives or sincerity of feelings each party may lay claim to. It emphasizes what individuals do, not what they say they mean. But the value of this approach should be judged on the proportion of patients who can be understood and successfully treated in this way when other approaches fail.

Other persons have been misled by the word 'games" and the ironic tone of clinical descriptions, and have considered this approach merely humorous. This is an error, in that both the intent and method are quite serious. As will be shown later, the analysis of games is not entertainment; it is an occasionally entertaining but serious and effective method of treatment.

Finally, it should be emphasized that it is not the intention of the descriptions given here to provide anyone with the possibility of name calling. For a doctor (or anyone) to point an accusing finger and say, "You're playing game X," can be merely destructive. The intention here is to heighten awareness of doctor–patient transactions so that diagnosis is improved, and so that doctors (and patients) do not let themselves get trapped into counter-productive relationships. Furthermore, becoming aware of the games played is an important part of the treatment process for the patient; name calling never is.

Research in this area is negligible, and we are almost entirely dependent on clinical observations and descriptions. An exception is the work of Bond and Pilowsky (10) investigating the relationships among subjective measures of pain in patients with advanced cancer, their requests for analgesics, and the medicating responses of the nursing staff. There were low correlations among the three variables. The subjective perception of pain by the patients did not always generate a proportionate request for drugs; requests when made did not consistently lead to the administration of drugs; and the strength of the medication was not proportionate to pain levels. Significant sex differences were noted, with the nursing staff tending to favor the female patients.

In a follow-up of these findings, Pilowsky and Bond (62) did a factor analysis of such transactions in a comparable patient setting. They found that the nursing staff tended to withhold the stronger drugs from the patients who had greater self-concepts of invalidism, but when such patients were women, the nurses more frequently took the initiative and medicated them with stronger analgesics. Older patients were likely to be given weaker medications.

Sternbach *et al.* (79) found that low-back patients, compared with arthritics, endorsed significantly more items on a questionnaire reflecting "pain games" being played with doctors, a result perhaps of the staff attitudes toward low-back patients.

Such studies as these are necessary to put a solid experimental foundation under descriptions of staff–patient transactions. It is quite important, in dealing with the difficult problems chronic pain patients present, that we have as objective data as possible.

THE BASIC PAIN GAME

As a result of a disease or injury, or of emotional conflict, a person experiences continued pain and gradually comes to think of himself as a chronic invalid and suffering person. This becomes his identity, and as with all of us, his actions and interactions are designed to confirm this identity (or self-concept). His interpersonal interactions take the form of games designed to maintain this identity, and a series of such games over time determines the individual's life-style. This life-style is as difficult to change as are those of alcoholics, addicts, or pious church goers (72,73).

The game begins when the pain patient sees the doctor and, stripped to its essentials, the following transaction occurs:

> *Pain Patient:* I hurt, please fix me. (*But you can't.*)
> *Doctor:* I'll fix you.

Procedures are performed; these fail, and relief is again demanded; the doctor admits failure, a referral is made and/or more procedures are performed, which fail, etc. The transaction is completed when the following exchange occurs:

> *Pain Patient* (in righteous indignation): Another incompetent quack.
> *Doctor* (defensively): Another crock.

This exchange occurs, with slight variations, in hundreds of instances every week in pain clinics around the world, and in thousands of doctors' offices.

The reason for this game, with its gimmick at the end where the patient triumphantly says, "Gotcha," can be described in several ways. In the existential model, the patient is simply making a statement about his identity, "I am a suffering person." Socially he is saying, "Look how much I suffer; you cannot diagnose my pain or relieve my suffering." At the psychological level, he is avoiding all intimacy and responsibility for his life, except to surrender to a surgeon for the sake of gratifying his body mutilation. At the biological level he can be said to be satisfying his needs for nursing care, for narcotics, and for sustenance through disability compensation (6).

How does this pattern develop? The prototype of such a transaction occurs in early childhood, to judge from the psychoanalytic literature (86). Here it takes the essential form of:

> *Child:* I don't feel so good.
> *Parent:* I'll beat you good, and then you'll feel something.

Later this pattern for masochism is reinforced with a variety of transactions which reduce to the following:

> *Child:* Beat me so I know you care (but you can't change me).
> *Parent:* I'll beat you and you'll be changed plenty.

This, of course, sets up the situation for the polysurgery addict, or for the pain patient, to say:

> *Pain Patient:* Fix me (but you'll fail).
> *Doctor:* I'll fix you.

In other words, in childhood the patient has learned that there is little affection at home, and in his need for this elemental feeling he has learned to substitute attention for affection. The attention comes either because he has pain, or it comes in a painful form. However, it is not necessary for the patient to have learned this paradigm in childhood, as a script for living. It is quite enough to have: (a) painful illness or injury; (b) unmet emotional needs, such as for affection; and (c) reinforcement of pain behavior through the full or partial meeting of these needs. These elements are enough to launch the patient on his new career or life-style as a pain patient. The life-style will continue until there are no more payoffs, and satisfactory alternatives are offered.

SOME SPECIFIC PAIN GAMES

There are a great many possible games involving pain, for after all they are a function of the patient's personality, his experiences, and his situation or circumstances. However, in dealing with a great many pain patients, it has become clear that certain themes and patterns recur between many patients and the persons who are important to them. These constitute some of the more common games, and their outlines here serve to illustrate the essential interactions and payoffs.

The Home Tyrant

A tyrant is one who gets his way with the aid of a weapon, and the patient's pain can be a powerful one. It can, for example, help him to get out of many responsibilities, and yet save face:

> *Pain Patient:* It's not that I don't want to (put out the trash, have sex, go to work). I can't.
> *Spouse:* That's all right dear. I understand.

The pain serves as an excuse with honor. Whoever would insist that the patient perform his responsibilities must be crass, unfeeling, and cruel. It is seldom discussed that the pain itself is not a disability, and that the word "can't" is inaccurate and really means "don't want to." Neither does the patient admit that since he is going to be in pain whether he lies in bed all the time or does what he normally would, he might as well get on with living; and since the patient does not say it, others do not either.

In addition to getting out of things he would rather not do, the chronic pain patient, by means of pain expression, gets others to do things for him. The expression on his face, his gasp, moan, or tears, cause concern, attention, and sympathy:

> *Pain Patient:* I hurt.
> *Spouse:* Shall I call the doctor (get your pills, take you to the hospital)?

Each of the spouse's offers are something the patient could do for himself. There is clearly more to the transaction than a simple request for assistance. It is both a reminder of the patient's suffering identity, and a regression to an earlier mode of behavior with overtones of magical thinking:

> *Child:* (Holding out injured finger.) It hurts.
> *Mother:* I'll kiss it and make it better.

The patient uses such a transaction not because it will relieve his pain, nor because he cannot phone the doctor himself, but because of the psychological payoffs. He gets sympathy, attention, and tender loving care, perhaps as he never got it before. Furthermore, he does not have to admit that he needs or wants these things (after all he did not ask to be in pain). He gets it all honorably. The problems this causes are basically twofold: (1) it reinforces the patient role, because needs are now being met which may go unmet if the patient improves; (2) it is very tough on the spouse, who has to continually be a parent to the childlike patient, and has no one to reciprocate.

The wielding of pain to elicit conforming behavior applies to the patient's children as well as his spouse. He can avoid disciplining them, yet can keep them in line by expressing his pain and producing guilt feelings in them:

> *Pain Patient:* I hurt.
> *Child:* I'm sorry I was noisy, I forgot.

Alternatively, the patient can be abusive to the children, and blame it on his pain which makes him very irritable:

> *Child:* I'm sorry I was noisy, I forgot.
> *Pain Patient:* When I get through with you, you'll never forget again.

In sum, the patient tyrannizes those at home by avoiding his responsibilities, controlling their behavior, and getting payoffs, while he lies around feeling sorry for himself.

Moral: Tender loving care is appropriate and necessary in the acute pain situation. It is inappropriate and destructive in the chronic situation.

CASE ILLUSTRATION 5

Mrs. F. B. is a 37-year-old housewife who is referred by a private neurologist because of intractable right occipital pain of about 13-month duration. She has been extensively evaluated, with apparently minimal physical findings to account for the pain.

Interview. Mrs. B. is a very heavy woman, who seemed to be in no apparent distress. However, she held her neck stiffly and did not turn her head much. Her manner was pleasant and cooperative, but at times she showed some irritation at certain questions.

Relevant History. Mrs. B. had a difficult early life, growing up in the Northeast. There were 11 children, and when her parents separated she and her twin sister went to a foster home until they were 9, then they went to an orphanage until they were 14. She worked through high school and afterward, then at age 24, she entered a convent for 1 year, leaving when she found it was not the life for her. She married her present husband when she was 27. Of her family, all still in the East, she is only close to her twin; the rest are like strangers.

Her husband is a career serviceman. They have two daughters, ages 8 and 3. The oldest daughter has cystic fibrosis. This is a very stressful situation. The patient's husband used to blame her for the child's illness, saying that because she carried the child, she must be responsible for the cystic fibrosis; he refused to accept responsibility for his genetic contribution. He has not raised this issue lately, however, and Mrs. B. says he has been "very good and helpful" in their recent move to this area.

The head pain began when Mrs. B., just home and convalescing from having her gallbladder removed, got up quickly to check her daughter's vaporizer unit one night, fainted, and hit her head on the corner of the dresser.

She takes a good deal of narcotics to control her pain, although she says they do not really do much good. She takes six Fiorinal and aspirin per day, and two Demerol and Dalmane at night (if her husband is home; otherwise she abstains from these at night in case she has to help her daughter).

Test Findings. On the Health Index, Mrs. B. endorsed a moderate amount of items relating to chronic invalidism and manifest depression, a significant amount concerning pain preoccupation, but no particular problems with doctors. The pattern suggests an asking for help in one who feels helpless.

The patient estimates the intensity of her usual pain as 75 on a 0 to 100 scale, which is severe pain. On the tourniquet pain test, her usual clinical pain level was matched at 5 min 47 sec, and her maximum tolerance was reached in 6 min 34 sec. Thus, her clinical pain is 88% of her tolerance, higher than her estimate of 75, and in the very severe range. This is rare in chronic organic pain states, and tends to occur most often in those whose pain is largely psychogenic.

The MMPI shows a distressed and hypochondriacal neurotic pattern which is classical for somatization reactions (Fig. 12). There is a great deal of somatic preoccupation, and denial of emotional problems, which serve to keep anxiety and depression within normal limits. However, there are signs that this pattern is not working entirely well as some agitation and depression are beginning to emerge. Her hypochondriasis and somatic complaints appear to be serving the function now of focusing her awareness away from other concerns.

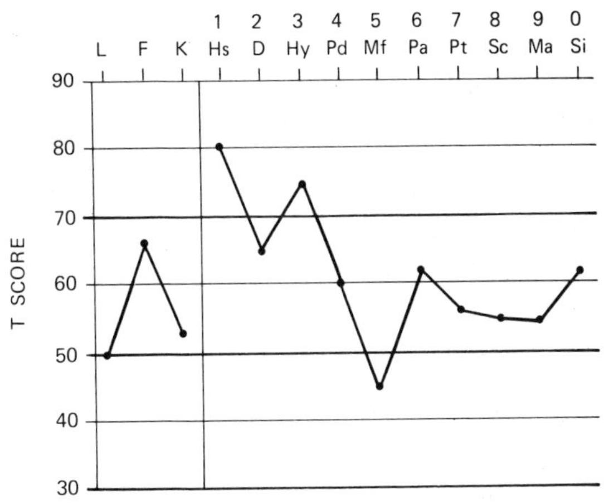

Fig. 12. MMPI profile of patient F. B.

Diagnostic Impression. Hysterical neurosis, conversion type (300.13).

Discussion and Recommendations. Mrs. B. is under a great deal of stress in caring for her sick child, and as time goes on she is approaching a tragedy. Her husband will soon leave for overseas duty and she will be facing the situation of caring for her child by herself. However, her husband has been of little emotional support to her, in fact, he has added to her burden by angrily accusing her of causing the child's congenital disease. It has only been since her accident that he has been helpful; she has now "got" him. It is quite likely that the accident and injury to her head gave her a kind of "time out" from her responsibilities, and satisfied her need to depend on her husband for a while. It is also possible that the patient hopes the service may see fit to keep her husband here since she, as well as the child, is ill. Thus, Mrs. B. really needs her "time out" on a long-term basis. Therefore, she continues to have her symptoms for psychological rather than physical reasons.

No further somatic diagnostic procedures should be carried out, as these only serve to reinforce the patient's idea that the real problem is physical, and in the absence of hard findings from all the exhaustive testing that has been done, it may now be safe to discontinue them. Mrs. B. should be told by the neurologist that there are no treatable physical findings, but that there are treatable psychological findings, and no matter what the original cause of the head pain, only the latter approach can now be expected to provide relief. Referral should be made to the psychiatric clinic for both individual and couples therapy. Mrs. B. should be tapered off her narcotics quickly, as she admits they do not help much, and she is probably addicted by now.

The Professional

The professional patient, like the professional athlete, is one who is paid for his role. The patient loses his amateur (acute patient) standing when he accepts financial reward for his patienthood. This may come in the form of compensation claims, litigation suits, unemployment benefits, welfare payments, social security disability benefits, etc.

The transaction begins with the patient presenting himself to the doctor with his various symptoms and signs:

> *Pain Patient:* Please fix me (but you'll fail).
> *Doctor:* I'll fix you.
> *Pain Patient:* How long before I can go back to work?
> *Doctor:* Not just yet—we'll see.
> *Pain Patient:* Sign here.

The professional patient seldom seems to want to avoid work. On the contrary, he acts as if the thing he wants most in the world is to return to work, and he is impatient with the doctor for restraining him. This occurs even when the patient has not worked in a number of years, and realistically cannot return to his former occupation. The tipoff to these patients is their refusal to seriously consider any other form of employment. They insist on wanting their usual work, and consider themselves disabled if they cannot perform their old job.

In fact, very few pain patients are totally disabled. They can always do something. It is not the doctor's job to find an alternative career for the patient—that is the patient's responsibility. If it seems realistic to the doctor that the patient cannot return to his former (usually laboring-type) job, he can set a time limit for the patient as follows:

> *Pain Patient:* Sign here.
> *Doctor:* O.K. I'm writing here that this is for 3 months only. By that time, I'm sure you'll have found some other kind of work you can do despite your pain. You're not totally disabled, you know.

CASE ILLUSTRATION 6

Mrs. R. D. is a 28-year-old housewife who was seen initially in consultation at a private clinic because of complaints of intractable head and neck and left arm pain of 2-year duration. This pain began with a whiplash injury following a rear-end auto collision, and was made more severe by a head-on collision 8 months ago.

Repeated neurological evaluations failed to reveal any significant findings, with the following exception: limitation of neck motion in all directions; generalized, nonradicular weakness of the left arm in the C5–C8 area; normal deep tendon reflexes; patchy sensory changes possibly greater in the C8 area; possible decreased strength in the left hand; tenderness and spasm in the left supraclavicular area.

Relevant History. The patient was born and raised in Houston, the youngest of three children. Her father, now 60, owns a car lot. Her mother, now 49, was a housewife, but with the children grown, now owns a dress shop to keep herself busy. The oldest brother, now 31, has an automobile paint and body shop, is married, and has three sons. The middle son, now 30, works for their father, is married, and has no children.

Mrs. D. says she was a "conceited brat" as a child, because she had her father "wrapped around her thumb"; she was "mother's baby," "teacher's pet," was smart (got A's) in school, and was popular. Her home life was (she says) very happy. She was double promoted in the second grade and finished high school at 16. She married at 17, and has a son now 10 years old. This marriage did not work out, she says, because she and her husband were both too young, and he continued to run around as if he were single.

After having been separated for about a year, they were divorced 6 years ago. At this time the patient saw a psychiatrist twice weekly for 6 months, because she felt "beaten down." The psychiatrist got her to see that her husband had done this to her and that he was the one who was at fault.

Four months after her divorce the patient married her present husband. He is the son of a famous musician and he himself had a musical debut when he was 9 years old. He attended college at various schools for 6 years but never completed work for a degree. After marriage, they both worked at record promotions and moved to New York where her husband was sufficiently successful to make commissions of $80,000 per year. However, Mr. D., now 29 years old, wants to become a millionaire by age 35, therefore he has begun to organize a new kind of promotion, and they have just moved to this area a few months ago. They will be leaving again in a few months. Mrs. D. says she is an active partner with her husband, making plans and decisions with him, making business calls around the country from their home, etc.

In addition to the neck injuries, Mrs. D. has had uterine difficulties; two cysts have ruptured and have caused peritonitis, and she has had numerous D&C's.

This seems to be a family problem, as her mother, all mother's sisters, and a cousin have had early hysterectomies. Mrs. D. is bitter about doctors telling her that there is nothing wrong with her and then having to be rushed to emergency rooms. She uses this argument, and others, to show that her neck spasms and tension headaches are purely physically caused and that there are no psychological factors. However, Mrs. D. admits that she was doing well until very recently when she played a game of tennis which resulted in severe pain.

There is also a problem with narcotic analgesics. The patient says she is allergic to all but morphine and possibly Demerol. Close questioning reveals that allergic reactions to each of a number of narcotics resulted in specific different kinds of rashes and other allergic responses, so this is apparently a genuine problem, and the nursing staff is kept running to give repeated injections of p.r.n. morphine.

An additional problem is that litigation from the auto accidents is still pending. Mrs. D., of course, denies any interest in these and even disclaims knowledge of their status, however, it is reasonable to infer some awareness of what is developing.

Test Findings. The patient estimates the severity of her pain as 95 on a scale of 0 to 100. This is the highest estimate that we have encountered and it suggests a dramatic complaint. However, it is confirmed by the ischemic pain test.

On the submaximum effort tourniquet technique, Mrs. D. matched the severity of her clinical pain at 12 min 42 sec, and her maximum tolerance was reached in 13 min 10 sec. Thus her clinical pain is 96% of tolerance, quite close to her estimate, and this suggests that it is very severe indeed.

On the Health Index, the patient did not show great amounts of chronic invalidism, manifest depression, nor pain preoccupation, however, she did show a great deal of anger and manipulative attitudes towards doctors, suggesting a tendency to play pain games.

The MMPI is entirely within normal limits (Fig. 13). There is evidence of a basically hysterical personality, with a tendency to somatization (conversion) reactions, with no evidence of anxiety or depression.

Discussion. The test results suggest that the patient has very severe pain which is primarily organic in origin, with only slight neurotic amplification. However, even apart from the neurological findings which suggest hysterically caused pain, there are reasons to doubt the test findings. These are: clear problems with narcotic analgesics; an excessive degree of anger towards doctors; the effect of pending litigation; and the exacerbation of pain by her own actions. All of these can account for her pain being more severe than it needs to be on purely physical grounds. Yet the patient insisted that her background was idyllic; her present circumstances virtually perfect; and she also refused to consider that there could be any psychological component to her pain. The patient refused

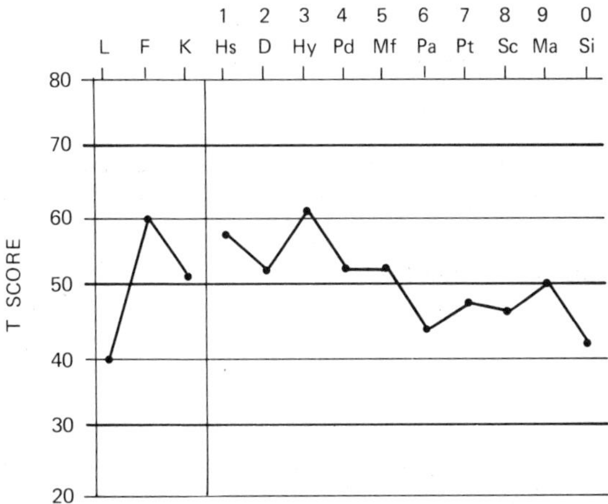

Fig. 13. MMPI profile of patient R. D.

transfer to the pain unit, and both the neurosurgeon and psychologist noted that her adamant stance was probably a pathognomonic sign of psychogenic pain, since patients with severe somatogenic pain are eager or willing to consider all approaches which could make the pain bearable.

A week after the initial consultation, Mrs. D. called and requested admission to the pain unit, saying she felt she could trust us. Her husband also called and arranged for us to meet together to discuss the unit and to have the program explained. Mrs. D., during the course of the introduction to the procedures, wanted to know what her games were, and we described the following: "Doctors have been wrong in the past about psychological problems so you must be wrong now"; "I have excellent insight from previous psychotherapy, and so I know there are no problems now"; etc. She said she was "offended" by this. However, she agreed that the process could be less painful than the headaches, that people can play games of which they are unaware, and that the process could help uncover problem areas such as sex, anger, or dependency needs. All this would be done while the surgeon reviewed her myelograms, pain medications were controlled, etc.

A few hours later, Mrs. D. checked out of the hospital, telling the nurses she did not like hospital rooms without carpets. The following week, a request for all records was received, since a court hearing was to be held on the first accident within a few days. Clearly, the patient's defensiveness and her behavior suggest a much greater case for psychogenic pain than was indicated by the psychological testing.

Diagnostic Impression. (1) Psychophysiological musuloskeletal disorder

(305.17), and (2) adjustment reaction of adulthood, posttraumatic neurosis (307.27), in an (3) hysterical personality (301.56).

The Addict

Very few patients are willing to admit to their need for narcotic analgesics. That is a privilege apparently reserved to professional drug addicts who begin their con game with that frank admission. (However, I have known true addicts who have feigned pain syndromes in order to get their drugs.) Pain patients express a horror at the idea of having to take medications on which they might become dependent, yet they maneuver the doctor into offering stronger analgesics.

Pain Patient: When the pain came on last night, I took the Darvon you gave me, and it didn't work, so I took some Talwin my neighbor had and some Codeine that Doctor Pushover had prescribed for me, and it only eased the pain a little bit. I hate taking all those pills. Can't you cut a nerve or something instead?

Doctor: I wish we could, but let's find a more effective analgesic since the others aren't helping you. You won't become addicted if you follow the directions.

After several such trials, the patient finds a certain drug which does the job. It not only eases the pain more than a little bit, but it makes him feel pretty good. The next transaction must ensure a steady supply.

Pain Patient: Doctor, this pain is excruciating, it's driving me out of my mind. Isn't there something you can do?

Doctor: Do you mean the pain's worse?

Pain Patient: Oh no, it's better now with that Percodan you prescribed, but I hate to take drugs like this. Can't you operate?

Doctor (relieved): No, I think we'd better just keep things as they are.

When the patient protests so much yet keeps taking analgesics, it is a good sign that an addiction problem is in fact brewing. There are several serious consequences for the patient, quite aside from any moral issues about taking pills to feel good. First, in chronic-pain conditions, physical tolerance to the drug develops, so that larger and larger doses, and stronger and stronger analgesics, are needed to produce the same degree of pain control. Ultimately nothing will work very well, and for the patient with chronic benign pain, with a long life ahead of him, this can be a significant problem.

Second, narcotics produce a physical dependency, so that not taking them results in withdrawal symptoms. Most pain patients do not experience typical withdrawal symptoms as do professional addicts, but instead experience a marked increase in their pain greater than that which they had before beginning to take the drugs.

Third, and related to the physical dependency, is the psychological conditioning which is established when pain signals are reinforced by analgesic intake. The continual pairing of pain and analgesic creates a psychological dependency, even though the patient may not be aware of any "craving." This conditioning is manifested by an increased level of pain whenever the patient "needs" his medication.

The evidence that these kinds of dependencies make patients' pain worse than it need be owing to physical reasons comes from studies of patients' pain levels when they are withdrawn from narcotics. An example, shown in Fig. 14, is provided by a Baptist minister who, as he put it, is "programmed to tell the truth." He was withdrawn abruptly from the narcotics that he took for low-back pain, and experienced a marked exacerbation in his pain, which subsided to a much lower level in a few days despite resumption of physical activities. This is a rather typical experience, seen in many patients. A different pattern occurs in patients who are withdrawn gradually. There is then no marked exacerbation, but the pain levels also fall gradually. Patients are usually quite impressed to discover that they have less pain despite less analgesic intake.

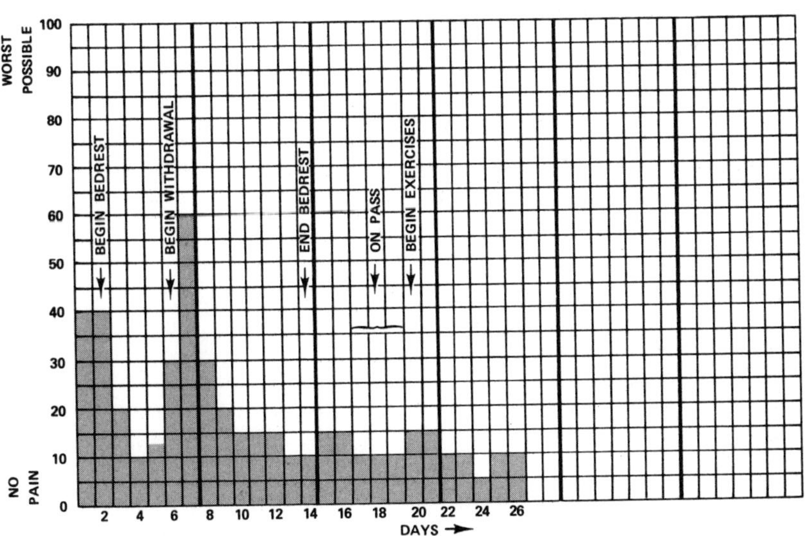

Fig. 14. Exacerbation and diminution of pain levels in a patient following abrupt withdrawal from narcotics.

For these reasons, and because only the salicylates presently are safe for long-term usage, the doctor must avoid letting himself get trapped by the patient who thinks he knows what is best for him.

Pain Patient: I hate taking all those pills. Can't you cut a nerve or something instead?

Doctor: I think you're right about those pills. They don't seem to help, and they'll only mess you up. Stop taking them.

Pain Patient: But what about the pain? It's driving me crazy, it's unbearable.

Doctor: You're just going to have to live with it. When it gets really bad, take one or two aspirins every 4 hours, no more.

CASE ILLUSTRATION 7

Mr. A. B. is a 38-year-old unemployed plumber who is seen on referral from the physician consultant to the narcotic treatment program. He had been placed on the methadone maintenance program for backache after his family physician had been instructed by the Federal Bureau of Narcotics and the State Board of Medical Examiners to stop giving the patient prescriptions for narcotic analgesics. The referring physician feels that the methadone has not proven to be of any value.

Relevant History. Mr. B. was married in 1956, at age 22, and was working as a plumber until he suffered a shoulder injury in an auto accident in 1959, the year his daughter was born. He has not worked regularly since that time (his wife works) because of the arm and shoulder injury. In 1962 he developed the low-back pain, and in 1966 began receiving narcotics for pain.

There are extensive workups in his chart, all with negative findings: from a neurosurgeon in July 1967, from a radiologist on a lumbar myelogram in August 1967, from a rheumatologist in March 1968, and another radiologist on a lumbar myelogram in March 1968, from another neurosurgeon in October and November 1969, and from an orthopedic surgeon in June 1972. There are other reports as well, none apparently finding any organic pathology.

Interview. The patient entered with an obvious chip on his shoulder. He defiantly asserted, without being asked, that no matter what anyone tells him, he will never believe that his pain is "psychosomatic." (In our experience, most patients with organic pain generators are willing to consider anything that might alleviate their pain, including looking into psychological problems. Those who most resist this approach tend to have the greatest psychological findings.)

Mr. B. quoted a local psychiatrist as assuring him, after one interview, that his backache was not "psychosomatic," and another unnamed psychiatrist was quoted as saying he would have to see the patient for a year to possibly give an opinion. However, the family physician states he has not received any psychiatric reports.

Mr. B. states that if any psychiatrist said the pain was "psychosomatic," he would have to prove it, and also prove what the patients' motives would be to have the pain. While this is relatively easy to do in Mr. B's case, this statement suggests his manipulation of doctors: the burden of "proof" is on doctors to show that he does not have pain, yet the patient has not done anything to get rid of his pain except to take narcotics—he has refused exploratory surgery and psychiatric treatment.

Mr. B. also implies blackmail: he states that he wants our reports in writing so that in the future, if pathology is detected, he can "come back on" the doctors who said there was nothing wrong, or that it was a psychological problem.

In addition to a sporadic work history for the past 13 years (he did not retrain or seek vocational rehabilitation), the patient has had a poor sexual adjustment for 10 years. When he does not take narcotics, his backache prevents him from having relations with his wife, but when he takes the drugs he is uninterested and/or impotent. (This is also atypical of patients with organic pain lesions.)

Mr. B. has been abusing analgesics for 6 years: morphine, Phenergan, Demerol, Percodan, Dilaudid, Talwin, and his favorite, Leritine. In addition to these prescriptions from his physician, at various times he would visit hospital emergency rooms to receive injections for the pain.

In addition to the challenge and threat mentioned above, Mr. B. presented in interview two other games: undiagnosable pain and unrelievable suffering—"You got to help me, Doc, it's your job (but you'll fail)"; and playing off one doctor's comments against another's—"Let's you and him fight."

Test Findings. On the Health Index, Mr. B. did not endorse a significant number of items relating to chronic invalidism, but did for manifest depression and pain preoccupation, and for problems with doctors.

This patient was seen before we had developed our technique of comparing the pain estimate with the tourniquet pain ratio. The ischemic pain test was done only to obtain a maximum tolerance time, to compare with others. Mr. B. tolerated the ischemic pain for 2 min, as compared to the average of 7 min for males with low-back pain.

The MMPI shows a quite depressed, passive, and dependent person with striking antisocial or sociopathic characteristics (Fig. 15). He has a great deal of hostility which is likely to show itself in psychophysiological symptoms and depressive affect, but without control factors, which are barely adequate, he could easily erupt into antisocial acts. Patients with this profile are typically found in medical clinics with persistent complaints which do not respond to treatment, and usually such patients have alcohol or addiction problems.

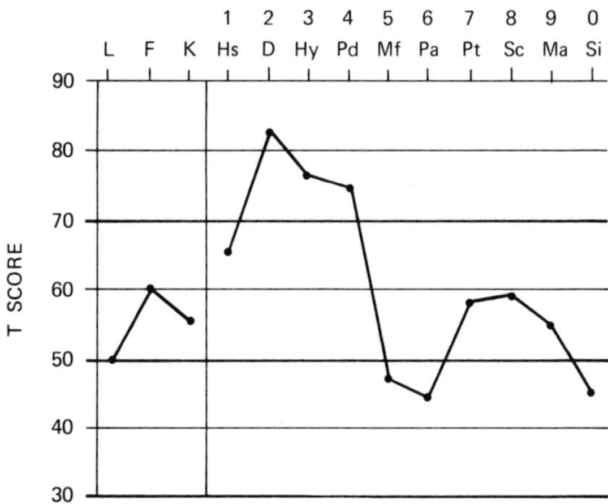

Fig. 15. MMPI profile of patient A. B.

Discussion. Although Mr. B. has not provided any physical pathology which could be treated, he has demonstrated psychopathology and psychological pain findings: (1) relatively low pain tolerance; (2) hysterical sociopathic personality characteristics and depressive affect, which may mask more severe psychopathology; (3) a history of sexual and work inadequacy and narcotic abuse; (4) a refusal to consider his psychological causes of pain; and (5) his playing typical games of painmanship with doctors.

Diagnostic Impression. (1) Depressive neurosis, moderate (300.47), in a (2) passive–aggressive personality (301.81), with (3) narcotic drug dependence (304.17).

Recommendations. Mr. B. must not be on any prescription analgesics. He must be told bluntly and finally that there are no physical findings to explain his pain, but there are psychological ones. If he hurts badly enough and cannot control it with an aspirin, he has the choice of bearing the pain or working to get rid of it in psychotherapy.

The Somatizer

In lieu of experiencing the pain in their lives, some patients experience (or focus on) the pain in their bodies. They insist that there is no problem at home, there are no stresses, they feel no anxiety, depression, or emotional upsets, there is no connection among (a) things happening in their lives, (b) their emotional reactions, and (c) their pain levels. They are, they believe, the embodiment of perfect mental health.

Doctor: I imagine this has been quite a strain not only on you, but on your wife too, and you've had to make some adjustments.

Pain Patient: I've been blessed with a very understanding wife, Doctor, and we haven't had any problems.

Doctor: But not being able to work, and all the visits to hospitals and clinics, and not sleeping nights. . .

Pain Patient: We've taken it all in stride, no problems. Of course I'm still trying to get relief, this pain never lets up.

Doctor: Have you noticed that sometimes the pain seems worse, when you're worried about things or you get upset?

Pain Patient: No, I can't say I have. I don't worry about anything. The only thing that bothers me is this pain.

Of course this bland denial of problems and worries may be accurate, but it requires verification. (My own experience is that it usually is a danger sign: it may predict the failure of any treatment–surgical, medical or psychological.) Verification of the patient's story means interviewing the spouse and patient together and inquiring of both of them how they have adjusted to their change in fortunes. There are usually financial, sexual, and mood changes which cannot have had no impact. If, in fact, these have not occurred, the patient is right and has no problem but his pain.

Usually the patient is merely blind. His family is suffering a great deal, and his somatization is merely a defense against his being aware of these problems himself, since he can tolerate physical pain better than he can emotional pain. The payoff, in other words, is the avoidance of facing the real-life pain by focusing everyone's attention on the physical pain. This is a very difficult gambit to counter.

Pain Patient: I don't worry about anything. The only thing that bothers me is this pain.

Doctor: But you have real financial problems, and your wife says you're very irritable, and she's getting pretty desperate.

Pain Patient: Well, if I could get rid of this pain everything would be okay.

Doctor: And if you can't, but have to live with it, how would you change things?

Pain Patient: I wouldn't change anything, we're really pretty happy.

Doctor: Then you have a rough future. You don't have any reason to get better.

Pain Patient: What do you mean?

Doctor: To get better, to overcome your pain, you're going to have to change yourself and make some changes in your life. But you seem satisfied with yourself and your life now, so why should you change anything? Why should you learn to overcome your pain when you already have everything you want?

Pain Patient: You see, it's not just in my back, but it goes down this leg . . . etc.

CASE ILLUSTRATION 8

Mrs. F. J. is a 50-year-old woman who is referred by a hospital psychiatrist because of complaints of several intractable pains. These are: (1) lumbar back, for 26 years; (2) thoracic back for 6 years; (3) right hand, for 10 months; and (4) right hip, for 4 months.

Interview. Mrs. J. is a cheerful, smiling, boyish-looking woman who seemed in no apparent distress. She is lithe in appearance, and although she shifted about a good deal in her chair, she got up and moved about very quickly and easily. She seems intelligent and well-educated, spoke articulately, and stated that she requested psychological consultation because extensive physical examinations failed to produce adequate causes for her pains.

Relevant History. Mrs. J. comes from a professional family. Her father was a civil engineer, her mother a social worker, and then a teacher. Mrs. J. was born in Mexico where her father was working, but returned to California as a small child. She has a brother, now 51½, a teacher, who has back problems also; he is married and has four children. Father died 7 years ago at the age of 72, of amyotrophic lateral sclerosis. Mother is alive at age 77, suffering somewhat from arthritis. When Mrs. J. was 13, her parents divorced. Father then left on a European trip and returned a year later with a Rumanian wife. Mother remarried to a Bulgarian when the patient was in her 20s, and the patient has a younger half-brother, now 35 and divorced.

In World War II the patient worked as a hospital corpsman in the service for 3 years, and injured her back. She had three operations, and when a fourth was recommended she refused it, became very depressed and suicidal, and entered psychoanalysis for 3 years, between the ages of 25 and 28. At this time also, she was working and going to college, and after some years finally became a physical therapist.

At age 37, she married an old family friend who had just recently been widowed. He was a public official 24 years older than she, now 74 years old. Since then she has not worked, but has kept house and has been very much involved in civic affairs. She felt she could marry this man because he did not seem to need to have children. He had been childless in his first marriage, and the patient had been warned, because of her back, not to bear children.

Mrs. J. feels that her health began to go bad 4 years ago following an airplane trip when she had a bad cold which resulted in an ear infection. (However, in that same year her husband developed heart problems and nearly died.) More recently, 4 months ago, the patient's right hip pain became a sudden and severe problem for no apparent reason, causing her to consult us. (Just 1 month earlier her husband had a hernia operation and has had an "irritable heart" since then.)

There are no clear physical causes for her hand and hip pain, no evidence of arthritis, fractures, etc. She has also had painful swelling of her feet, tiredness, rashes, etc. In the past she has injected IM Talwin, but her analgesic intake now is Tylenol #4 (1 gr. of codeine) five times daily.

Test Findings. On the Health Index, Mrs. J. endorsed a significant number of items relating to chronic invalidism, manifest depression, and pain preoccupation, but no significant number concerning problems with doctors. The pattern suggests a self-concept of sickness and suffering.

The patient gave two estimates of the severity of her pain, on a scale of 0 to 100. Her pain lately has been 60; at its worst, it has been 80. However, on the tourniquet pain test, her current clinical pain level was matched at 30 sec, her worst clinical pain was matched at 2 min 20 sec, and her maximum tolerance was reached in 7 min 23 sec. Thus her current pain is only 7%, her worst pain only 32%, of her tolerance.

This discrepancy is significant: she estimates her pain to be in the moderate to severe range, but it is in the trivial to slight range. The difference may be considered to be the amount of "neurotic overlay," or at least, the extent of her problem of communicating accurately.

The MMPI was almost invalidated by Mrs. J.'s attempt to portray herself as the picture of mental health (Fig. 16). With her intelligence and sophistication, this may be not merely a defense against recognition of internal conflicts, but a quasideliberate attempt to appear conventional and virtuous to others. In fact, she overdid this test-taking attitude and so presented herself as a self-righteous person without even the minor faults most persons admit to. This caused her to receive somewhat reduced scores on the clinical scales. Nevertheless, the profile is one of a woman with a very strong potential for conversion reactions. There is a great deal of somatic preoccupation and hypochondriacal concerns, and a very

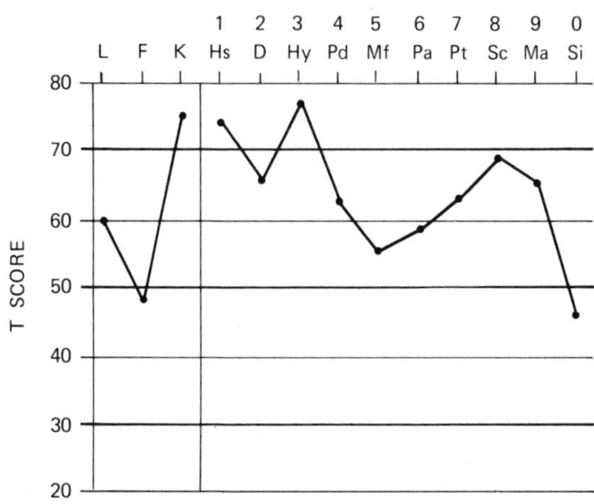

Fig. 16. MMPI profile of patient F. J.

great amount of denial of awareness of psychological problems. This serves to keep depression and anxiety within normal limits, but it is at the price of having to focus a great amount of attention on physical complaints. There is evidence as well that she may be experiencing some symptoms of a thought disorder, and that her somatizing defenses are either masking a more serious emotional disturbance or are strained by current stresses at home.

Diagnostic Impression. Hysterical neurosis, conversion type, (300.13).

Discussion and Recommendations. Mrs. J's history suggests that her recent pain episodes have come in close association with her husband's serious health problems. The psychological test results support the idea that her symptoms can be explained on psychological grounds alone. If there were physical findings as well, then the psychological test results would predict a significant "functional overlay."

More important than the determination of cause is the selection of treatment. It seems that Mrs. J. has thus far failed to provide her physicians with any organic pathology which they can treat, and so she has looked to the psychological approach. There is some psychopathology which can be treated, and this may indeed provide her with pain relief.

The area of difficulty which seems to be suggested by the interview and tests, is her relationship with her husband, and the anxiety produced by the threats to his health. The difference in ages, previously unimportant, is now becoming significant, and Mrs. J. may now be going through some internal struggle related to her personal and sexual relationship with him. Inasmuch as Mrs. J. did well in psychoanalysis many years ago, it is reasonable to predict that she would do well again in psychodynamic psychotherapy.

There seems not to be a good justification for the strong narcotics she is taking. Her pain is not great by any means, and with continued use her dependence on narcotics is very likely to increase the severity of her pain. In the absence of clear organic pathology, Mrs. J. should not be dependent on any prescription analgesic. She should be able to get by on aspirin or acetaminophen.

Follow-up. Mrs. J. declined to consult a psychiatrist, and instead sought treatment from an acupuncturist, who she felt was benefiting her.

The Confounder

For some patients the payoff for painmanship is not money, drugs, or avoiding emotional upsets, but confounding the doctor. This is particularly worthwhile the more specialized or famous the doctor is. Every pain clinic has encountered patients who express respectful disappointment with the great medical centers where they have been treated in the past. Their records show good initial responses to the several kinds of therapy they have received, then a return of the pain. No surgery, medication, physical therapy, or psychotherapy has helped for very long, but initially all did. By their initial favorable response to treatment, the patients seduce the doctors into pursuing the full course of treatment, then utterly defeat them.

With this kind of history, the doctor should be forewarned, but he usually takes the bait anyway.

Pain Patient: I'm sure happy to be accepted here, Doctor. This is the most wonderful program I've ever seen. The other patients tell me how much they've been helped, and I'm beginning to feel really hopeful. You people sure know what you're doing.

Doctor (embarrassed): I'm glad of that, and I hope we can come up with a solution for you.

Pain Patient (3 weeks later): Doctor, this stimulator you implanted is perfect. This is the first time in 11 years I've been completely free of pain. I don't know how to thank you.

Doctor (pleased): That's very good news.

Pain Patient (2 months later, tearfully): Doctor, the pain is back and it's excruciating. Can't you do something?

Doctor (flustered): I'm not sure. We'll have to admit you again.

With the history from the old records, it should be obvious what is happening, and only a hard line can stop this game. This is done by predicting it.

Pain Patient: I'm beginning to feel really hopeful. You people sure know what you're doing.

Doctor: Thank you, but I'm not hopeful at all. In fact, your case is almost hopeless. If you get better, it will be due more to your will power than to anything we can do. If you don't get better, I won't be surprised, considering your history.

Pain Patient: (3 weeks later): I don't know how to thank you.

Doctor: Don't thank us. What did we do? You helped yourself. And we'll see if it lasts. Don't forget your pain has always returned before. Whether it stays away now is entirely up to you. I'm skeptical, but we'll see.

Another way of forestalling the Confounder's game is to give patients the opportunity of choosing which "diploma" they will earn (see Fig. 27, Chapter IX).

CASE ILLUSTRATION 9

Mrs. S. W. is a 53-year-old housewife who is seen because of intractable rectal pain of $2\frac{1}{2}$-year duration. She has numerous other medical complaints, including diabetes which is currently being evaluated at a private clinic.

Mrs. W. was previously seen by several physicians in this city for the rectal pain, then at the Mayo Clinic, then at this hospital a year ago, with a staff conference review. Apparently all reports are of negative findings except for her complaint of pain, and all recommendations have been for the patient either to live with the pain, or to obtain psychiatric treatment for what seemed to be a depressed state. The patient chose the former course, but recently, while at the private clinic for control of her diabetes, she was referred to the pain clinic because of her continued complaint of rectal pain.

Interview. Mrs. W. was accompanied by her husband, who is 58. She is a rather open and friendly woman, who got emotional when discussing the incident that initiated this problem (she became very angry) and when discussing the absence of their sex life since that time (she became very tearful and self-reproachful.) Her husband in contrast is a dour and resentful-looking man, who bitterly emphasized their mistreatment by the medical profession. Both of them openly admitted to being very bitter about their experience lately; whenever they digressed, they returned to examples and generalizations about raw handling by doctors. Mrs. W., in particular, seemed anxious to know whether I believed her story. She occasionally joked and slapped my arm in a friendly way. She was not in any obvious distress except for some slowness in sitting down and getting up. However, she later called me to say she'd been in great pain, but had been hiding it.

Relevant History. The patient grew up on a dairy farm in the Northwest, the youngest of three girls; she has a sister 5 years older and one $1\frac{1}{2}$ years older, both are married and have children, and all are living in the home town. When Mrs. W. was 37, her mother, at age 60, died of a CVA. Three years later, her father died, at age 62, of cancer of the pancreas. She continues to be on good terms with her sisters and their families, and sees them often on visits.

Mrs. W. was the only one of her family to leave the home town, because her husband was a career officer in the armed service. He retired 15 years ago at age 43, after 23 years in the service, because of chronic ulcers due to the stress of his job (personnel work.) After doing some real estate sales and industrial engineering, he took a civil service job, which he still has, collecting fees at the trash dump not far from their home. They need the extra income because of their medical expenses, and he also wants the extra group medical insurance coverage in addition to that to which they are entitled because he is a retired career serviceman.

The W.'s have been married for 31 years. They have three children: a daughter, 36, a housewife in the Midwest with five children; a daughter, 29, a housewife in this city with one child and another on the way; and a son, 25, who works as a police officer, married with one child. He left the parental home finally (after being in the service, then getting more schooling) to get married about 3 years ago. By that time Mrs. W. was working part time in a local cleaning establishment in order to have something to do.

Then, $2\frac{1}{2}$ years ago, Mrs. W. was in a local hospital for an anal fissure repair, when postoperatively a nurse attempted to give her an enema without the syringe tip on the tube. This caused excruciating and violent pain and rectal tearing. Her physician assured her she would heal; she did not. He said he would complain about the nurse; he did not. She continued to be in pain. Finally, she and her husband complained to the hospital and their physician discharged her from his care. They sued the hospital, but "records were forged" and they lost. Other doctors refused to accept her. Finally one repaired her, but the pain persisted, and the saga continued to the Mayo Clinic and then here.

The story is nearly incredible, yet plausible. The description of her agony is given with great vividness and affect, though it has been told often. It could have happened, yet their difficulties with physicians "eight or ten times" since then suggests that there is much more going on. The patient is particularly bitter that the same nurse is still working at that hospital, although she has made "other mistakes" since then. Mrs. W. says she feels strongly that she needs to protect her children (!) from this sort of thing. The feeling of the need for revenge comes across very strongly.

She currently takes a barbiturate to get to sleep at night; APC with codeine, two–eight tablets per day; and 5 mg of diazepam twice daily.

Test Findings. On the Health Index, Mrs. W. endorsed a very high proportion of items defining chronic invalidism (seven of ten), very few for manifest depression (four of twenty), an average number for preoccupation with pain (five of ten), and very many for being involved in pain games with doctors (eight of ten). Thus, this test confirms the impression from the interview that the patient sees herself as a chronic invalid whom doctors do not take seriously.

Mrs. W. estimates her rectal pain to average about 40 (moderate) on a scale of intensity of 0 to 100, although it varies from 25 (slight) when resting to 80 (severe) when long on her feet or after defecating. This average of 40 suggests she is not often in great distress.

On the tourniquet pain test, she tolerated the arm ischemic pain for 14 min 30 sec, a high tolerance level, even taking into account that the dominant arm was used instead of the nondominant arm because she could not get a ring off an arthritic left knuckle. Her usual clinical pain level was matched at 11 min 0 sec. This is 76% of her tolerance, much higher than her estimate of 40.

There is clearly a discrepancy between her estimate of the severity of her usual clinical pain, and the matching of the ischemic clinical pain levels. Usually the latter is more accurate and reliable. In this case, the former is probably more to be believed, because she seemed in no distress when stating the ischemic pain equalled her clinical pain, nor indeed when she stated she had reached the unbearable level.

The MMPI profile shows a somewhat conventional and virtuous self-appraisal almost to the point of defensiveness and self-righteousness (Fig. 17). She is basically an hysterical personality who focuses on numerous somatic complaints as an aid in denying emotional or interpersonal discontent. At present her attempt at such denial is strained, and she is showing signs of a mild to moderate agitated depression. There is some slight tendency to a thought disorder which is probably secondary to the agitation, and a fair amount of suspiciousness and resentment which is a part of it. The overall picture is one of a somatizer who is now agitated in reaction to a current illness or situational difficulties.

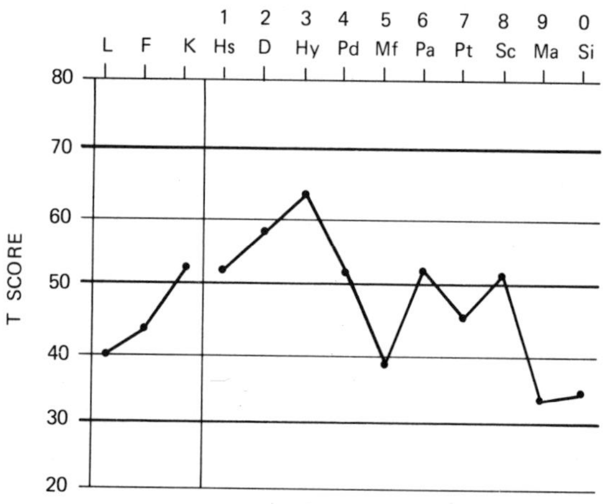

Fig. 17. MMPI profile of patient S. W.

Diagnostic Impression. (1) Depressive neurosis, mild (300.46), with agitation, in an (2) Hysterical personality (301.56).

Discussion and Recommendations. Mr. and Mrs. W. seem to have turned in upon themselves since their last child left home. The patient's illnesses have become the center of their lives, and they are almost totally preoccupied with her health. They have no sex life, virtually no social life, and little to do except brood and worry about her. When they do leave home, it is to venture forth into the now dangerous enemy territory of doctors' offices and hospitals. They now collect grievances quite bitterly and guard themselves against incompetent, unethical, and greedy doctors by seeking second opinions, etc.

It seems obvious that the two of them constantly reinforce each other in this behavior. It is like a *folie a deux* which borders on the delusional. The patient no doubt has medical problems, but they do not seem exotically unmanageable. What is intractable is the complaint of pain. With this symptom the couple can prove how incompetent physicians are, and how much Mrs. W. suffers and is wronged.

Treatment must consist of couples therapy, as well as antidepressant medications for Mrs. W., because unless Mr. W. can participate in the joint venture of initiating a new and more satisfying life-style, her improvement will founder on his sour resentments.

PLAYING GAMES VERSUS TREATMENT

Anyone familiar with the works of Potter (64) and Berne (6,7) will have no difficulty in recognizing and countering the moves of any pain patient. This is easy to do, and it is usually enjoyable. And after one has treated a hundred or more patients, there are few surprises left, although occasional new twists and puzzles appear. However, as we pointed out earlier, merely naming the patient's game is not helpful, and is potentially destructive.

Similarly, merely countering the patient's games is not necessarily therapeutic; it is easy enough, but does not by itself help the patient to acquire more adaptive behaviors. To be effective, any maneuver must take place within the context of a total treatment program whose goals and methods are explicit and agreed upon in advance. We will describe these procedures in detail in Chapter IX. The point is made here because the game aspect of the overall treatment program is often the most intriguing and fun, and it can be overemphasized to the detriment of actual treatment.

What is useful about the game approach, especially when it is taught properly to patients, is that all parties learn to pay more attention to what they actually do, rather than to what they intended, said, or wished. (The doctor also finds himself under some scrutiny in this respect, and if he is honest enough he soon learns from the patients if he has been playing games with them.) By examining the discrepancies between intentions and behaviors, by making explicit the self-defeating actions which have been automatic and unrecognized, the patients for the first time have the opportunity to make deliberate choices about how they will live. If a person must live with pain, he can do so as a chronic patient, or he can seek satisfying alternatives.

It is clearly helpful to a patient to find out that he has been making his family miserable, if he hasn't realized it. It is also helpful to him if his family learns that it is possible to talk about it in a constructive way, that they need not feel guilty and need not tolerate tyrannical invalidism, and that for their part they can help the patient meet his needs by reinforcing constructive behaviors rather than his sick role.

Similarly the patient is helped by learning how to talk with doctors. It comes as a revelation to most patients to learn how certain things they say or do are red flags to surgeons, for example. And it is sobering to a pain patient to have his fellow pain patients tell him he is getting a lot of mileage out of his complaints. The patient who adamantly insists on total relief of pain, when it cannot come to pass, can at least learn that he has company, and that some of that company have learned to get more out of life than he has (30).

These are some of the uses of the analyses of pain transactions, within the setting of a total pain treatment program; a fuller description is given in Chapter IX.

VIII

Diagnostic Procedures and Predictions

In this chapter on how to diagnose patients in chronic pain, we draw on the information presented in the previous chapters. That information, from clinical studies and objective research, may be summarized *very* briefly as follows.

The complaint of pain, by itself, is about as likely to be a sign of mental as of physical disorder. If it is a mental disorder, it is most probably a neurotic one, and it is equally likely to be a reactive depression or anxious hysteria. These are the most common diagnoses in psychogenic pain (although patients with schizophrenia or endogenous depression may occasionally present pain complaints). On the other hand, patients with somatogenic pain lasting many months or longer develop hypochondriacal and depressive features which make them seem to be neurotic, much like the psychogenic pain patients. Further, many chronic pain patients engage in game playing as part of their attempt to adapt to the pain experience, and in this respect seem to have a personality disorder as much as do alcoholics or drug addicts.

Accordingly, it would seem to make good sense to provide chronic pain patients with both a psychological and physical workup. The physical, particularly neurological, examination, of course, is quite routine and virtually never omitted. However, the psychological examination is usually deferred until it is fairly certain that no organic explanation of the pain is forthcoming. In other words, psychological (or psychiatric) referral is made only after excluding physical causes, and thus tends to be reserved for psychogenic pain patients.

This typical process has certain drawbacks. For one, it deprives the somatogenic pain patient of a psychological diagnosis and the appropriate psychiatric treatment. The assumption is made that if an organic lesion is present, and it is consonant with the nature of the pain complaint, then that lesion is a full and adequate explanation of the complaint, and no psychological problems are involved. Of course the facts, as we have reviewed them, indicate otherwise. Indeed some of the evidence suggests that when psychological problems are treated, the pain due to physical lesions often becomes quite bearable.

The other major drawback to the traditional diagnostic procedure is that it also penalizes the psychogenic pain patient. He is so diagnosed, as we have said, by exclusion of physical findings, and then referred for psychiatric consultation. Unfortunately, unless the consultant has specialized in pain patients, he will find no obvious pathology in his mental status examination, and will refer the patient back; this is particularly likely if there are minimal physical findings as in low-back strain, scarring, or "adhesions" from previous operations.

Much of the problem in making psychological diagnoses in pain patients is that most consultants have not had a wide experience with such patients, do not know what to look for, and because the referring physician has not asked a very helpful question (it is usually, "Psychogenic pain?") the consultant tends to look for an either/or answer. He is thus easily persuaded by the patient that the pain is "real" and "physical." The psychological consultant, for example, sees that the patient is oriented and has no obvious thought disorder; therefore he is not psychotic and the pain is not part of a somatic delusion. The patient denies any problems at home, but admits to being irritable and depressed because of the pain; therefore he is not showing *la belle indifference,* is not an hysterical denier, and the "appropriate affect" suggests the patient is not particularly neurotic. Thus the absence of apparent psychological findings causes the patient to be referred for further physical examination, and so it goes, back and forth, with treatment delayed unnecessarily.

It is the purpose of this chapter to specify some of the diagnostic procedures which are helpful in outlining the nature and extent of the psychological problems. This will include both objective test data and clinical interview material. The purpose of the diagnostic procedure is to answer these questions:

1. Why is this patient in pain (if there are no obvious physical findings)?
2. Why cannot this patient live with his pain (if there are known physical findings)? What makes it worse than it need be?

PAIN LEVELS

First in importance, and especially helpful to those who must manage the patient's care, is some assessment of the severity of the patient's pain. It is no good being stampeded into a surgical procedure, or prescribing potent narcotics, for the palliation of a pain which turns out to be slight or trivial in intensity, but which perhaps frightens the patient. To rely solely on the patient's verbal description of the intensity of his pain is to invite contamination from such personality traits as bodily preoccupation, anxiety, and degree of extraversion, and from such cultural factors as permitted expressiveness—as we have previously described. The result of all these influences may be an overly stoical patient forced to suffer needlessly, or an overly expressive one made to go through unnecessary procedures.

It has previously been shown that individuals can assign numerical values to painful stimuli in a reliable and lawful way, using several different psychophysical methods (77). It seems reasonable to expect that patients can do as much for their clinical pain levels, as normal subjects can for experimental pain. The author has found it helpful to use and compare two methods.

Magnitude Production: The "Pain Estimate"

The simplest procedure is to have the patient assign a number to the intensity of his pain, on a scale of 0 to 100. Almost everyone is familiar with percentages, and this scale presents no difficulties. The instructions are:

> We need to get a more accurate idea of how severe your pain is. On a scale of 0 to 100, in which 0 is no pain at all, and 100 is pain so severe you'd commit suicide if you had to endure it more than a minute or two, what number would you give your *average* pain? What is your average pain *these days*?

Defining a score of 100 as "suicide" has proved necessary because some very dramatic patients have said, while seeming calm and relaxed, that they were experiencing a pain of 100, some even said it was 110. By insisting that this could not be, else they would not be sitting there, they were persuaded to give a more accurate rating.

The number the patient gives is a form of magnitude production. This number is recorded, to be compared with a value from an ischemic pain test (magnitude matching) to be described below.

In our treatment program, patients record these pain estimates each day, assigning a value at the end of the day to what they consider to be the average pain for that day. From these data we may obtain some idea of the reliability and the validity of this measure. Figure 18 shows the pain estimates for all the patients (about $\frac{1}{3}$ of the total) who received neurosurgical treatment. The relative constancy of the pain levels for the first 4 weeks, prior to surgery, attests to the reliability of the measure. The marked decrease following surgery is an index of the measure's validity, in that it reflects the expected effect of the intervention.

By way of comparison, the daily pain estimates of an individual patient who did not receive surgical treatment, was shown in Fig. 14 in the previous chapter. That graph reflected an increase in pain with the sudden withdrawal of narcotics.

From these figures it is apparent that the pain estimate, as simple and as subjective as it seems to be, reflects something valid about the patients' pain

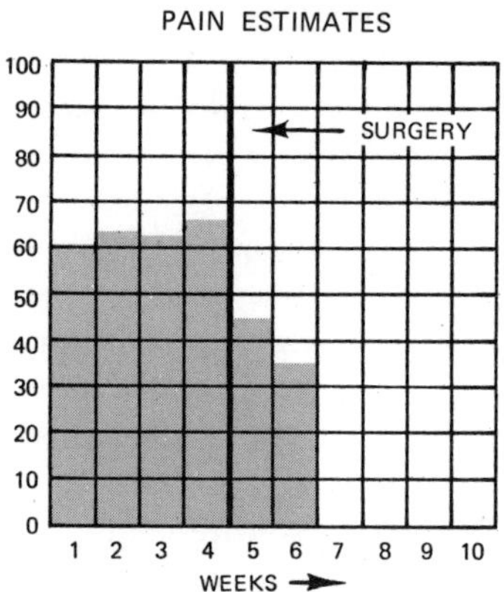

Fig. 18. Pain estimates of 25 patients who received surgical treatment for various organic pain syndromes. Each bar represents an average of seven days' estimates, averaged across all patients.

level, in that it seems to vary in the appropriate direction reflecting the interventions which are made. And the consistency of the measure in the absence of (preceding the) intervention speaks well for its stability or reliability.

Magnitude Matching: The "Tourniquet Pain Ratio"

It is possible that the pain estimate may be as much loaded with psychological and cultural influences as are verbal descriptions of pain levels. It is therefore helpful to introduce a painful physical stimulus against which the patient may match his clinical pain level. This would not eliminate the subjective response, but the introduction of the painful stimulus into the patient's judgment, for comparison, should make the measure of clinical pain more accurate. In general, magnitude-matching procedures are more precise than magnitude production.

There are a variety of experimental pain measures which can be used, and the results from several techniques are rather similar (94). Some workers have insisted that it is essential to use a quantifiable stimulus, as in electric shocks or radiant heat, but this is arguable. We do not bother with such refinements, for example, when taking a patient's temperature or blood pressure. What is necessary is to have a method which is simple and convenient to use in an outpatient clinic or at the patient's bedside, which can be shown to be valid and reliable.

In our program we have adapted the submaximum effort tourniquet technique, developed by Smith *et al.* (66–68). In addition to having the practicality desired, it mimics the duration and severity of somatogenic pain, and even in experienced subjects with little anxiety it produces the marked autonomic changes which frequently accompany pain of pathological origin. In the studies by Smith *et al.*, validity is supported by the responses of the ischemic pain measure to various analgesics, and reliability by the authors' replication of results.

The essence of our method is that blood is drained from the nondominant arm by means of a tight rubber bandage, which is removed after a blood pressure cuff is inflated well above systolic pressure. The patient then squeezes a hand exerciser slowly 20 times, and a stopwatch is started. The patient reports when the pain equals his usual clinical pain in intensity (even though it may be a different kind of pain). Then the cuff is left on until the patient reports that the pain is the maximum he can tolerate. These two times, the clinical pain level and the maximum tolerance, are recorded.

We have previously reported the excellent reliability of this method (75). If no intervention occurs (surgery, psychotherapy, changes in analgesics), replicability of the times is on the order of 0.8, which is not merely highly statistically significant, but very reliable.

The tourniquet pain ratio score is computed by dividing the time to reach the clinical pain level by the time to reach the maximum tolerance, and multiplying the result by 100. This gives a score comparable to the pain estimate, such as 45, or 60, and this score can be compared with the patient's pain estimate. Note that this tourniquet pain ratio is not dependent upon a comparison of the patient's pain threshold or pain tolerance with that of a standardization group. Group measures tend to have very great variability, and it is not very helpful to know that a patient is more or less sensitive or tolerant to pain than are others. The tourniquet pain ratio gives a more meaningful score, namely the relationship of a patient's clinical pain level to the maximum he can tolerate. In this connection the tourniquet pain ratio seems somewhat related to what Wolff (91) has called the pain endurance factor.

The validity of this ratio score can be indicated by the changes in this measure which reflect what is done to the patients. In Fig. 19, the tourniquet ratio score is shown for the same group of patients whose pain estimates were illustrated in Fig. 18. In our program, the ischemic pain test is performed once a week on each patient; he matches the pain level with what he considers to be his average pain for the preceding week. It can be seen that there is good stability of these scores prior to surgery, and that they then reflect the effects of the pain-relieving procedure.

A somewhat different pattern is shown by those patients whose treatment does not include neurosurgical procedures. These patients' tourniquet ratio scores are illustrated in Fig. 20. Here it is seen that the scores rise with the passing weeks, after an initial drop, with a marked increase in the final week. The cause for this seems to be a decrease in analgesic intake, and the marked

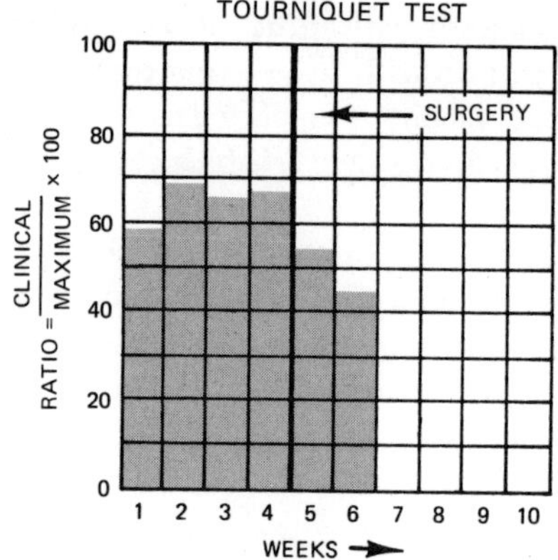

Fig. 19. Tourniquet pain ratio scores of 25 patients who received surgical treatment. Ischemic pain tests are performed once weekly. Compare with pain estimate scores in Fig. 18.

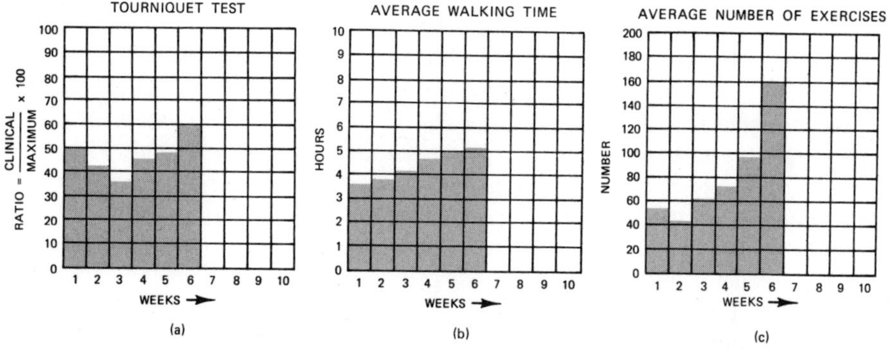

Fig. 20. (a) Tourniquet pain ratio scores for 50 patients participating in treatment program, with no surgical intervention. The rise in pain levels closely parallels (b) the increases in walking time, and (c) the number of exercises performed.

increase in activity levels as reflected in the time the patients spent walking and the number of exercises they performed.

From these changes in tourniquet ratio scores—the decrease with neurosurgery for pain relief, the increase with increased activity level—it is obvious that the scores reflect changes which are not merely reliable, but valid indicators of pain as well.

As previously stated, we obtain both scores from patients. Neither score correlates with any personality variable, nor does the difference between the two (75). Patients typically estimate a higher pain level than that which they give by matching, and occasionally the difference is quite marked. It has been found helpful to draw a "pain thermometer" and present it to the patient. If the difference between the two scores is great, he is asked why he thinks it is; the explanation can reflect the patient's neuroticism, or expressive style, or some other factor of diagnostic value. An example is given in Fig. 21, of a patient who estimated his pain at 85, but whose ischemic pain test showed that his clinical pain level was only about $\frac{1}{3}$ of his tolerance. His explanation of the difference consisted of a lengthy discourse on his accident and operations. Test findings and interview confirmed a suspicion of extreme hypochondriasis and passivity.

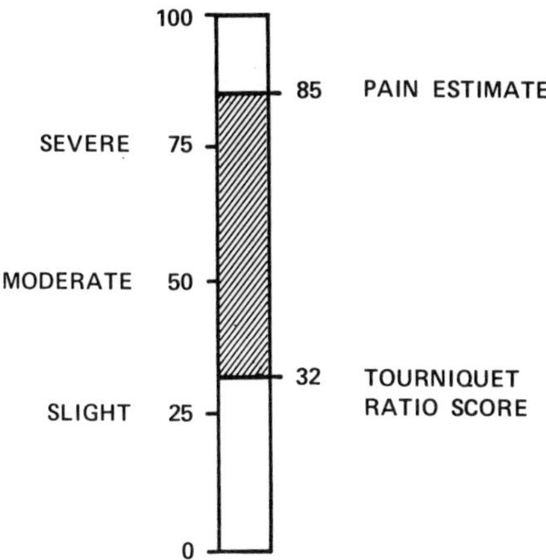

Fig. 21. Differences in two pain scores of a hypochondriacal patient with low back pain and clear physical findings.

It is clear that a procedure such as described has great advantages over the reliance on purely verbal descriptions of the severity of pain. In particular, it has proved to be a helpful instrument for a doctor to use in being firm with those patients who insist their pain is agonizing but whose tourniquet pain ratio scores are considerably less than their verbalized estimates. When they say, "Doctor, you don't know how terrible this pain is!," we are sometimes able to say, "Yes we do, and it's not that bad." We have been able to save a number of patients from the potentially damaging effects of their own bad judgment because of this procedure.

PERSONALITY TRAITS

There are essentially two ways of assessing personality, by test and by interview. Either method will provide the necessary information for making a diagnosis and outlining the psychodynamic mechanisms. The interview has the advantage of providing a "flavor" of the patient, and of establishing a relationship which is helpful in initiating treatment. Furthermore, when one knows what to look for, the interview technique can be quite brief. We have many times been able to confirm Engel's (23) observation that the necessary information can be obtained in from 30 minutes to 1 hour.

The psychological test, particularly objective tests rather than projective ones, is less personal, but has the distinct advantage of providing quantitative information. This is necessary for measuring both the effect of treatment on a particular patient and the overall effectiveness of the treatment program.

Accordingly, we have found it helpful to combine the two approaches, administering both a psychological test and a clinical interview, finding that the information obtained from each supplements the other. The test provides data for evaluating outcome effects, as well as diagnostic information. The interview allows for the gathering of personal information, evaluating of personal style, and the negotiation of a treatment contract.

Psychological Test

To be useful, an objectively scored test must be valid, reliable, and easily administered. In the United States, the most widely used test by far is the Minnesota Multiphasic Personality Inventory. It has a truly voluminous literature, and is composed of items which differentiate among various psychiatric groups and normals. The average patient usually takes about 2 hours to answer the 566 true–false statements, and scoring can be done by hand or computer to yield profiles as illustrated in previous chapters.

The test has disadvantages in that it is somewhat ethnocentric and age specific. Not everyone, for example, knows what is meant by, "I used to like drop–the–handkerchief." Nevertheless its popularity is due in large part to the fact that there are validity scales which measure test-taking attitude, and that the clinical scales conform relatively closely to the psychiatric nomenclature.

For our purpose, the test is helpful in providing measures of hypochondriasis, depression, and hysteria (the "neurotic triad"). Different scale configurations, as well as absolute scale scores, carry different diagnostic implications. In general, the highest score seems to be the one most likely to reflect the patient's subjective complaints, while diagnosis is dependent upon the overall configuration of scores. In Fig. 22 we show four profiles most commonly encountered in chronic pain patients. It should be noted here that these profiles are common in most chronic diseases, and are not pain specific. They can be found, for example, among patients with multiple sclerosis and arthritis. Furthermore, the profiles do not permit differentiating psychogenic from somatogenic patients, since as we have seen the two groups tend to look psychologically similar. However, our experience permits some remarks about the clinical characteristics of pain patients who show these profiles as illustrated in Fig. 22. It should be pointed out that these profiles have not been systematically cross validated on a new patient sample, and so they are suggestive only.

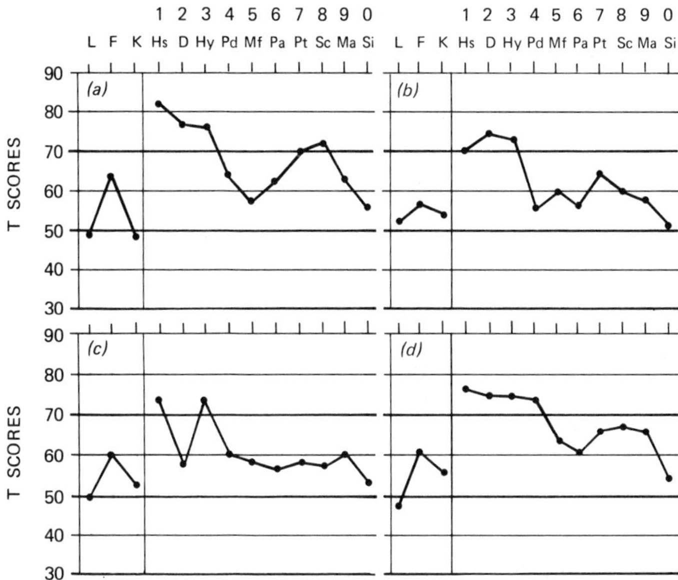

Fig. 22. Some typical MMPI profiles in chronic pain patients. (a) Hypochondriasis; (b) Reactive depression; (c) Somatization reaction; (d) Manipulative reaction. See text for details.

Hypochondriasis (Fig. 22a). Not only is the Hypochondriasis score the highest in the profile, but it is above the T score of 70. In this pattern, somatic preoccupation is extreme. To obtain such a pattern, the patient has to endorse a great number and variety of bodily complaints, including very many that would be totally unrelated to his specific pain problem. This profile seems somewhat more common among the somatogenic than the psychogenic pain patients.

As illustrated in Fig. 22, the profile is a composite of 15 patients who were judged "failures" of our treatment program, i.e., although they may have reported lesser degrees of pain than on admission, they continued to return to clinic after discharge with obvious signs that their pain was still the central factor in their lives. Patients with such profiles, and an organic generator for their pain, are most likely not to benefit from treatment, as they cannot for long ignore their symptoms, even when these are slight and not surgically correctible. These findings are similar to those of Pilowsky (59), who found that poor treatment outcome in hypochondriacal patients was associated with organic pathology, among other variables. He also found that older males and younger females did less well in treatment.

Reactive Depression (Fig. 22b). This profile is associated with the subjective experience of depression, and although the patient may insist it is in response to living with pain, he nevertheless is willing to admit that the pain has gotten him down. It is more common in the somatogenic pain patients, and more than the other profiles it is likely to be associated with a good premorbid adjustment. In our experience, whenever the Depression score is at or above a T score of 70, the patient is likely to show a favorable response to antidepressant medication; this is particularly so when it is also the highest score in the profile.

The profile shown in Fig. 22 is a composite of 15 patients who were clearly "successes" of our treatment program. On follow-up clinic visits they not only continued to report significantly lowered pain levels, but no longer sought relief and indicated they had more important things in their lives to enjoy. Thus this profile of reactive depression responds readily to treatment, and, in fact, may be considered to predict success. Pilowsky (59), also found that anxiety and depression correlated with a good outcome in hypochondriacal patients.

Somatization Reaction (Fig. 22c). This profile is so consistently associated with somatic complaints in psychiatric patients that it has been nicknamed the "conversion-V" and the "psychosomatic-V" pattern. It consists of both somatic preoccupation and the use of hysterical denial of psychological or interpersonal problems (assuming that the Hysteria score is not elevated because of the endorsement of items which also are part of the Hypochondriasis scale.) In this pattern, it appears the patient focuses on his physical symptoms in order to avoid awareness of latent depression, which is repressed.

However, although the pattern may predict conversion or psychophysiological symptoms in a psychiatric population, and may, in fact, be more common among psychogenic pain patients, it is also quite common in medical and surgical populations, and occurs frequently in somatogenic pain patients. Among the latter it seems to indicate that the patients have learned to live with their pain by deriving satisfactions from the invalid role. This is different from the hypochondriacal reaction, in which the patient is constantly worried and preoccupied with his symptoms, is forever finding new ones, and does little else but notice and catalog them. In the somatization pattern, the patient focuses almost exclusively on the single pain symptom, indicates that the rest of his life is just fine, thank you, and will the doctor be good enough to eliminate the pain.

In our program we have had moderate success with patients showing this profile. The patients have already made the first steps toward their adjustment, although it may not be a very satisfying one. Most of such patients find it possible to enrich their lives at least moderately, to become less symptom centered, and thus on follow-up do not seem to demand relief of unrelievable pain, i.e., they are further along in their adjustment.

Manipulative Reaction (Fig. 22d). We are coining this diagnostic term to represent the "con artist." The profile shown here is a composite of only 6 patients, but they were consummate game players who fooled the staff (and patients) in our treatment program. Each of the patients had clear physical findings, and there was no question of malingering in the usual sense. However, they persuaded us to perform unnecessary operations, or write narcotics orders, or sign disability claims, and only long afterwards did we learn directly from the patients what they had done and why.

The characteristic of this profile is that the Pd (psychopathic deviate) scale is elevated nearly as high as the neurotic scales. This Pd scale represents anger, manipulativeness, acting out, etc., and when it is as high as Hypochondriasis and Depression, it is a good bet that the patient is going to use his symptoms and signs quite deliberately and consciously to get something he wants. Lest it be thought that this profile is based on too small a number to be significant, it turns out that a very similar profile appeared in a larger series of low-back patients who had litigation pending (80), shown in Fig. 23. Fortunately, the proportion

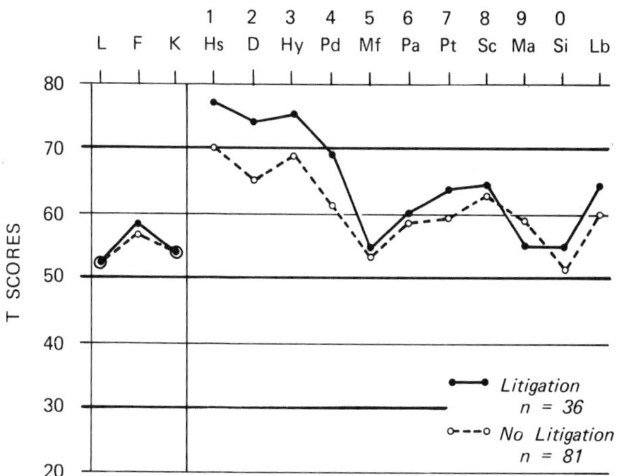

Fig. 23. Comparison of patients with low back pain who had some form of litigation pending (lawsuit, application for social security, or welfare or unemployment benefits, etc.), and those who had never initiated such action or whose application was settled. The "litigation" group has significantly higher elevations on the neurotic and Pd scales. (After Sternbach *et al.*, 1973, reproduced by permission of *Psychosomatics.*)

of patients who present with this profile is small, and one could exclude them from a treatment program as soon as it became apparent that their behavior was confirming the prediction made from their test profile.

Predictions. Although it is premature to be confident of predictions in the absence of cross-validating data on large numbers of patients, there are certain suggestions which emerge from our small scale retrospective study. In general, if a treatment program wants to obtain an impressive record of success, it will screen patients and accept only those whose profiles show either reactive depressions or somatization reactions. Contrariwise, a program whose patients have mostly hypochondrical or manipulative reaction profiles will probably compile a miserable record. In between, with good moderate success, will be those programs which take in all applicants who meet other requirements.

Interview

The advantages of the interview are that it provides the interviewer with an awareness of the patient, due to the immediacy of his presence, which cannot be obtained from any test report, no matter how thorough and eloquent. It provides the opportunity to obtain historical information from the patient, and to inquire how the patient met, and meets, various stresses. Finally, it provides the opportunity to assess what the patient needs and wants and how to tailor the treatment program to his needs, i.e., to engage him in a treatment contract.

The way to assess the patient's personal style in the interview is to observe *how* he interacts, as well as what he says. Does the patient whine or demand, or seem surly or flattering, for example? What emotional response does he elicit from the interviewer—admiration for bravery, sympathy for suffering, irritation for trivial complaints, boredom, etc.?

In addition to this interpersonal style, there are some facts which are important to know, involving three major areas of the patient's life. (1) Who is at home? How do they react to (what is the impact on them of) the patient's pain? What has happened to the patient's sex life as a result of the pain? (2) What work does the patient do? How have fellow workers and bosses reacted to the patient's pain? If he does not work, what does he do for income? (3) What is the patient's history with respect to pain medications?

Notice that these are different from the questions usually asked in the psychiatric interview. Usually, the interviewer would inquire about what was going on at home or work when the pain came on, i.e., he would seek to establish significant antecedent events as possibly causative. Furthermore, there is often an attempt to uncover something in the patient's childhood relationships which seem to have laid a pattern for the present behavior. We have found, however, that a past–present linkage is helpful in traditional psychodynamic psychotherapy, but less useful than a present–future linkage in our brief treatment program. The information we have found most helpful is not so much what precipitates or exacerbates the pain, but what are the payoffs or consequences of pain. Particularly with patients whose pain is clearly somatogenic, and whose problem is one of learning to make the best of it, information about the effects of their pain behavior is particularly important.

The reason for this, as Fordyce *et al.* (25,26) have shown quite convincingly, is that the consequences (reinforcers) of pain behavior can serve either to maintain and enhance the behavior or to extinguish it. When patients are being seen diagnostically, it is presumably because their pain is being maintained against their wishes. The maintenance occurs because certain needs are being met by the reinforcers. The diagnostic problem, therefore, is to determine the consequences or effects of the pain behavior, and from these one is able to infer which needs of the patient are being met and by what reinforcers. Treatment would consist of helping the patient to obtain these by healthy or adaptive behaviors, rather than by pain or other maladaptive behaviors.

With respect to these payoffs the patient receives, it is sometimes helpful to ask the patient what he would lose if he did not have the pain. Almost everyone who has had to accommodate to chronic pain will lose something in the process of readjustment if the pain were removed. Going over the patient's typical day in some detail will reveal those present rewards which would be lost.

In addition to the home relationships, including sex, and the work problems, it is important to learn specifically whether there is litigation involved, or some form of financial compensation which the patient risks losing by getting better. This is a most difficult area, in my experience, because the "compensation neurosis" does not yield easily to treatment. The details of the patient's sources of income are quite important to know, as is the patient's willingness to risk this income by getting better.

It is also important to know all the medications the patient has been taking, and all he has tried in the past. It is helpful to ask which of the pills seems to do the most good, i.e., which is the patient's favorite or which he seems to depend on or need. Addiction problems are quite common in pain patients, and one should be particularly concerned with the narcotics, barbiturates, and hypnotics the patient uses.

Finally, it is helpful to ask the patient how he would live if he could get rid of his pain. What is it he would do that he is not doing now? The way in which this question is answered (realistically or unrealistically, with bewilderment, with indifference, etc.) carries some diagnostic value. And the content forms the basis for the treatment contract.

Predictions. The kinds of information described above tend to be qualitative rather than quantitative, although it is possible to construct rating scales on which interviewers could agree with a good degree of interrater reliability.

Nevertheless, on the basis of clinical experience, it is possible to predict which patients with chronic pain will do well in a treatment program, and which will not do well.

In general, patients who are married and have family support tend to do better than those who have never married, or who are formerly married but living alone. Patients whose sexual adjustment was good prior to the onset of pain tend to fare better than those whose sexual adjustment was poor or marginal. Patients who have continued to work at their occupation, or who have retrained themselves to work at a less demanding job, do better than those who have not worked for some period of time, and both of these groups improve more than those who are supported by disability, unemployment, or welfare benefits.

Patients who have tried prescribed analgesics, found they did little or no good, and stopped taking them, tend to do well in treatment. Patients who have become iatrogenically dependent on or addicted to narcotics do less well, but can be helped, whereas those who, once introduced to the drugs, quickly and persistently have abused them, tend to have a more difficult time in treatment. The poorest prognosis tends to be associated with drug addiction prior to the onset of pain, and with alcoholism. Most of the patients displaying the manipulative reaction, in fact, were alcoholics who also abused drugs.

Psychologists and psychiatrists will recognize that we are describing criteria similar to the good versus poor premorbid adjustment criteria that have been developed for psychiatric patients. It was not so intended, but, in fact, most of our "failures" have been loners or have had poor marital adjustments, have been living on disability or welfare income, and have abused alcohol or drugs for some time. On the other hand, most of our "successes" have been well and happily married, have been either working or living on *savings,* and have had no addiction history. It has been common to hear these patients say, of the potent analgesics, "I don't think they really help that much. They just cloud my mind, and I'd rather not take them." None of the "failures" have ever said that.

Clearly, treatment programs which have limited resources, and which must screen applicants, could probably get best results by concentrating on those patients whose premorbid adjustments were good, in the senses mentioned. However, it should be remembered that these descriptions are of clinical impressions, and other centers will wish to acquire their own criteria, hopefully employing more quantitative measures as predictor variables than we have.

Fordyce (personal communication, 1971) has also evolved a set of predictors for his behavioral pain treatment program, which he considers tentative rules of thumb. Positive indicators are: (1) pain problem several months old; (2) patient rests to ease pain, activity worsens pain; (3) patient on p.r.n. pain medications; (4) pain has gradually worsened or spread over time; (5) patient is capable of walking (except for pain or disuse); (6) pain is possibly greater than it need be on physical grounds. As general negative indicators, he lists pain which awakens the patient at night, or is sporadic with days or weeks between bouts of pain, or pain which is proportional to the organic lesion.

These characteristics clearly have to do with the ready availability of operant pain behavior which can be shaped in a treatment program, and represent additional characteristics which can be used for prediction or screening.

IX

Treatment Methods and Evaluation

Although it is convenient for descriptive purposes to separate the assessment and treatment processes, in fact they shade into each other, and it could be said that treatment begins as the patient considers the answers to such questions as, How would you like to live if your pain were less? What would you lose? etc.

Many patients have never seriously considered the possibility that they may have to adjust to their pain. It is as if the time they have spent in pain is suspended time, that it does not count against their life span, and when relieved these patients expect to start again in life where they left off, even though many years may have elapsed since they were pain free.

The introduction of realistic goals, and a contingency plan if surgery is not feasible or is unsuccessful, is often the first step in treatment and is the essence of the treatment contract. Patients who can have successful pain-relieving surgery must prepare to return to a life which may have become foreign to them, much as repatriated prisoners of war must expect a serious readjustment process. And those patients for whom surgical pain relief is not possible must plan to reenter their lives in spite of their pain.

THE TREATMENT CONTRACT

There is always a treatment contract, a fact often overlooked by many physicians, even though it may be only implied. The patient always has certain expectations of the doctor, and the doctor likewise has certain expectations of the patient. Most often these are never verbalized, and consequently the implicit expectations affect the doctor–patient relationship without much awareness by either party. In most acute situations it does not seem to matter. But in dealing with chronic pain patients, who have usually (by definition) been to many doctors and have obtained inadequate relief, keeping the expectations implicit can invite a great deal of mutual exasperation as the two parties work at cross purposes.

The treatment contract should be explicit and specific. Ideally, nothing should be left unsaid about either the goals or methods of therapy. However, it is more often than not a characteristic of pain patients, with their somatizing life-style, that they tend to be practical and action oriented rather than imaginative and verbal, and so, in practice, it often takes days or longer for them to be able to bring out some of their concerns. Thus, the interviewer must abandon the traditional nondirective role, and be as active and assertive as necessary to learn from the patient what the patient wants in the contract.

It is best to begin at the beginning rather than take certain assumptions for granted. Does the patient want to get rid of, or significantly reduce, his pain? Is he willing to work at this problem? He must say "Yes" explicitly to both these questions or there is no point in proceeding (76).

We do not let the patient give an affirmative answer to these questions glibly, pointing out that he probably has very good psychological and/or physical reasons for having the pain, that it now obviously plays a very significant role in his life, and that it will take a lot of work, courage, and adjustment on his part to either give it up or overcome it. We add that it is unlikely, by the time the patient has gotten to us, that there will be a simple remedy which will abolish the pain, but that he and we may learn how to reduce it significantly.

At this point the patient usually thinks we are accusing him of malingering or imagining the pain. He acquires a stiff demeanor and begins a recitation of his history, symptoms, and findings, including the contradictory information he has been given by various physicians and surgeons. The patient's message is that (a) doctors cannot be trusted, (b) he has proof to counter our insinuation that the pain is "all in his head," and (c) he expects us to take away his pain magically, and conceives of his role as one of passively acquiescing in allowing us to fix him.

We stop this by making these implications explicit, and point out that, of course, he will be worked up for possible neurosurgical or other somatic treatment, but that the odds—by his history and our own statistics—are 2:1 against his obtaining such relief. We do not accept patients with psychogenic pain, and ours is not a psychiatric service. Is the patient willing to work to get rid of his pain? It often takes several repetitions to conclude these preliminaries with an affirmative answer from the patient. There is the passive–aggressive ploy, "I'll do anything you say, Doc." It can only be countered by, "I'm not saying anything, just asking." There is the setting–us–up gambit, "You're my last hope (only suicide is left)." We give the responsibility back to the patient, "No, you are your own hope. Do you want to work at getting better?" And so on. Only when a game-free willingness to work at treatment is expressed can we continue.

The next step consists of determining in specific detail how the patient would wish to live if his pain were gone or significantly reduced, and of considering whether all his needs would be satisfied if these goals were achieved. Concurrently, we consider what the patient would be giving up if he gave up his pain, i.e., the current satisfactions he risks losing.

When asked how they would live tomorrow if their pain were relieved today, almost all patients say they want to go back to work. This is automatic, as though they have often been accused of trying to avoid work and so need to assert their honest intentions. It often turns out that what they mean is to go back to their pre-pain occupation, even though this may be totally unrealistic in the face of their actual physical disability (apart from the pain) and in view of the number of years that have gone by since they worked.

We react with incredulity and ask for an explanation. It is not so much that we question the patient's motivation, as his judgment, (but the motivation too is a little suspect, else the patient would have found a way to work if he wanted or needed to). Inevitably the patient will describe how difficult it is to make ends meet on his meager disability income, how ashamed he is that his wife is working or that they are living on welfare, or perhaps how boring it is to sit around home with nothing to do. We argue with each point: he may need an increased pension to live better, but not a job; lots of wives work; welfare was made for just such cases as his; he may just need a hobby not to be bored; etc. We wonder whether he really took satisfaction from work, or if it was something he resented but felt forced to do.

The reason for our taking the part of devil's advocate in this transaction is that we want to be sure that the patient's goals are not only realistic, but genuinely motivated, that he really wants these things. If we have settled on a specific job as his first goal, such as, say, half-time television repair work, then we go on to a next goal, inquiring what he would do for fun, relaxation, or hobby. We question and challenge this too, until we are sure he wants none, or comes up with something about which he can get enthusiastic and which is also realistic. These goals, regarding work and play, should ring authentically from the patient, and the interviewer should be suspicious of half-hearted ideas suggested by the patient because of assumed expectations of the interviewer or of "people."

Surprisingly, often we have to raise the question of the patient's interpersonal relationships, for he seldom explicitly states this as a goal for improvement. Yet often he is clearly lonely—never married, divorced, widowed, or in an unsatisfying relationship, and with no close friends. Sometimes the patient hints at a strained relationship: "I'm the luckiest man alive that my wife is so understanding"; or, coolly, "Sure, we get along."

In this area the interviewer must press more gently than with respect to goals for work or fun, but he must press nevertheless. Patients will naturally be more defensive about such personal matters, and the interviewer will need to show understanding of how it is frequently easier to tolerate physical pain than the pain of loneliness, rejection, or heartbreak. But why cannot the patient get and remain close to others? How are his needs for company and emotional "stroking" being met? Is he really content with being a "loner"?

And so it goes for each goal, examining the extent to which needs are being met, and the realistic changes in his life which the patient would like. As a minimum, the interviewer should be sure to cover the areas of work, play, and personal relationships, because these are basic for all persons, and it is highly likely that the patient's pain is at least potentiated by lacks in these areas, or reinforced by his satisfying such needs with his pain behavior.

Once specific goals are obtained, we may have a list which looks like this:

1. Do small appliance repairs in my home, to supplement welfare income,
2. play cards once a week with neighborhood friends,
3. improve relationship with wife—fewer fights, better sex life.

These goals were obtained from a former laborer who initially insisted he wanted to return to physical work (despite a bad back), and that he had no problems other than his pain. The interview developed that he did nothing but sit around at home getting on his wife's nerves, that he had no social life at all. These goals were elicited from him, and he seemed quite pleased with them. He thought his life could be much more satisfying if he could attain them.

Of course, it is not reasonable to expect anyone to achieve his new life's goals quickly. However, it is possible to break down the attainment of each goal into discrete, step–by–step activities which, over time, lead to the attainment of the ultimate goal. Thus, the next step is to specify the activities in which the patient must engage to bring himself closer to his objectives, and the things which the staff will provide to help him. These represent subcontracts for attaining subgoals. For example, the patient will have to attend a shop program in the hospital, or a training course in a local school, to learn small appliance repairs, and the staff will help him locate the appropriate program. He will have to inquire of his neighbors to find which of them would like a regular evening of cards. And he and his wife will have to attend some counseling sessions to discuss and resolve their problems. We find it important to write all these details out, so that both the patient and the staff are clear as to exactly what is expected and that no misunderstandings develop. An example of such a contract, from our inpatient Pain Unit at the Veterans Administration Hospital, San Diego, is shown in Fig. 24.

The importance of this written contract, besides making the treatment plan explicit, is that it recruits the patient into an active partnership in his treatment. A patient is too often willing to be a passive reporter of his history and

TREATMENT PLAN

NAME: K.R. No.

I WANT TO ACHIEVE THESE GOALS:

1) LEARN WOODWORKING, SET UP SHOP AT HOME
2) WORK OUT MARITAL PROBLEMS
3)
4)

TO ACHIEVE THESE GOALS, I WILL:

1) WORK IN HOSPITAL WOODWORKING SHOP
2) INCREASE ENDURANCE FOR STANDING
3) ATTEND COUNSELING SESSIONS WITH WIFE
4)

TO HELP ME ACHIEVE THESE GOALS, STAFF WILL:

1) PROVIDE TRAINING IN WOODWORKING
2) PROVIDE PHYSICAL THERAPY + MEDICATION CONTROL
3) PROVIDE GROUP THERAPY + MARITAL COUNSELING
4)

K.R.
(Patient)

RAS
(Staff Member)

OCT. 11, 1972
(Date Today)

Fig. 24. A sample "contract", or treatment plan, showing patient's goals and his and the staff's obligations for achieving them.

symptoms, and a doctor is too often willing to think of the patient as the passive recipient of surgery and medications. But the patient who is actively engaged in his own treatment, who each day makes a little more progress towards the goals which will satisfy unmet needs, is in fact slowly weaning himself from dependence on doctors and hospitals.

Goal-related behaviors in general are inconsistent with the pain state. When these pain-incompatible behaviors are experienced they expand the time the patient spends in a nonpainful state. For example, if the patient is engrossed in learning how to fix a toaster, or if he is having sexual relations, he is not having a pain experience, or at least certainly not showing pain behavior. Patients typically report they are not aware of their pain at such times, or that it may be there but that it does not bother them.

Therefore, after drawing up the contract, we instruct the patient in how to build up his tolerance for his desired activities. If he can only work in the shop for 30 minutes before his pain becomes severe, then he should start with a 15-minute session and then quit; then the next day for 20 minutes, and so on, adding 5 minutes each day, until he has reached his goal of the amount of time he wishes to spend. Similarly, if he can only sit to play cards for 1 hour, and he wants to enjoy a 4-hour card session, then he can start on the ward with a 45-minute session, and each day increase his endurance by 5- or 10-minute intervals. There is a risk involved in gradually increasing the time spent in pain-incompatible tasks, in that the patient stands to lose some of the gratifications obtained through pain behaviors before there are adequate gratifications from the goal-related behaviors. Therefore, we encourage the patient to "fake" not having pain initially as he embarks on the difficult and unaccustomed first steps toward healthy behavior (76).

OPERANT CONDITIONING ON THE WARD

While the ultimate goal is to abolish or diminish the patient's pain experience, one of the intermediate methods is to modify his pain behavior. This is not for the purpose of producing stoicism in the face of suffering, but because, in fact, changes in behavior are followed by changes in experience.

The principles of this method were described by Fordyce *et al.* (25) and may be summarized as follows:

1. Behavior is governed by its consequences. Those consequences which increase the probability of occurrence of a behavior are called positive reinforcers, and those which decrease its probability are called negative reinforcers.

2. Pain behavior, whether verbal, motor, or physiological, is but a subclass of behavior generally, and like all behavior it can be maintained, enhanced, or

extinguished according to which reinforcers a patient receives for his pain behaviors. Positive reinforcers are usually attention, sympathy, concern, analgesics, and rest. However, for some it is isolation or restless activity that may be reinforcing.

3. To extinguish pain behaviors, withhold the positive reinforcers when these behaviors are emitted. Instead, give the positive reinforcers immediately when the patient engages in the pain-incompatible, goal-related behaviors which have been specificed.

In practice, it usually develops that pain behavior is maintained or enhanced by attention, rest, and analgesics. For example, if a patient is lying quietly in his hospital room, he is likely to be ignored by the busy nursing staff, and he will begin to feel lonely and miserable and his pain will get worse. Pretty soon he will cry out, and immediately he will receive nursing attention, and perhaps medication. Thus, his pain behavior is positively reinforced, and is more likely to recur. As a consequence of this conditioning process, he will both experience and express more pain when next he needs company or medication.

The operant conditioning approach on the pain ward is designed to reverse this procedure. Nursing staff praise the patient's initial goal-directed activities, and notice and compliment progress. Sociable conversations are held whenever patients are engaged in pain-incompatible activities. On the other hand, pain behaviors are ignored, so that if a patient complains of pain, or requests medication, the nurse may look out the window, yawn, or walk away. Similarly, analgesics are administered at regularly spaced intervals so as to break the associative link between the experience of pain and the need for the drug, and doses are gradually reduced.

Of course, this procedure must *never* be used with acute pain patients: such patients need to regress, and deserve sympathetic attention for their pain, and hospital personnel need to know when and how much the patients hurt. It is also unethical to manipulate patients' behavior without their knowledge and consent. In our program, patients are told what to expect from the nursing staff and why, when the contract is made, and several times during the course of their stay the principles described here are discussed in group therapy, using patients' experiences as specific examples.

The effectiveness of this approach is dramatic, and if one is a pragmatist, that is justification enough for following such a mechanistic-seeming procedure. We have seen several patients, who had been bedfast for many weeks, walking a mile a day within 3–4 days, attributable to little else than nurses' expressed delight with their first tottering steps. We have also reported more systematic results (30), showing that, in general, patients' pain estimates decrease or remain at the same level despite evidence from the ischemic pain test that actual pain levels may also be increased due to the increased activity.

As our treatment method is not "purely" an operant one, the evidence from Fordyce *et al.* (26) is more convincing. Using only the operant techniques described, uncontaminated by group therapy, and with a population of patients whose surgical histories are very impressive, these authors show clearly how

DAY OF WEEK: THURS. DATE: NOV. 2, 1972

	SITTING		WALKING & STANDING		RECLINING	
MIDNIGHT	MAJOR ACTIVITY	TIME	MAJOR ACTIVITY	TIME	MAJOR ACTIVITY	TIME
12 - 1					T.V.	60
1 - 2	TALKING	60				
2 - 3					SLEEP	60
3 - 4					"	60
4 - 5					"	60
A.M. 5 - 6					"	60
6 - 7			CLEANUP	60		
7 - 8	TALKING	60				
8 - 9	BREAKFAST	60				
9 - 10	GROUP	60				
10 - 11			SHOP	60		
11 - 12			SHOP	60		
NOON 12 - 1	LUNCH	60				
1 - 2			SHOP	60		
2 - 3			SHOP	60		
3 - 4			SHOP	60		
4 - 5			CLEANUP	60		
P.M. 5 - 6	SUPPER	60				
6 - 7					T.V.	60
7 - 8					"	60
8 - 9					"	60
9 - 10					"	60
10 - 11					"	60
11 - 12					"	60
TOTAL TIME		6 HRS.		7 HRS.		11 HRS.

0 10 20 30 40 50 60 70 80 90 100

NONE — X (at 80) — WORST POSSIBLE

AVERAGE PAIN FOR THE DAY

Fig. 25. Sample of daily log kept by patient, recording various activities and average pain estimate for the day. These logs form the basis of patients' graphs of their progress, and of program's evaluation of its effectiveness.

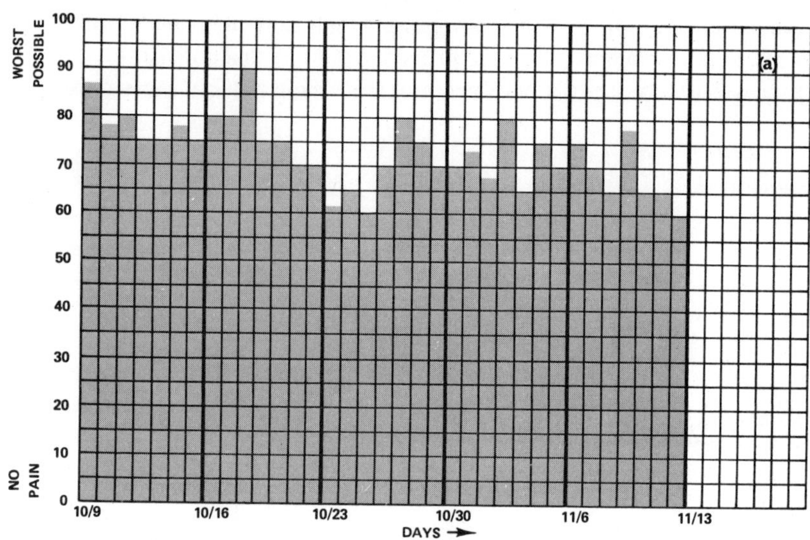

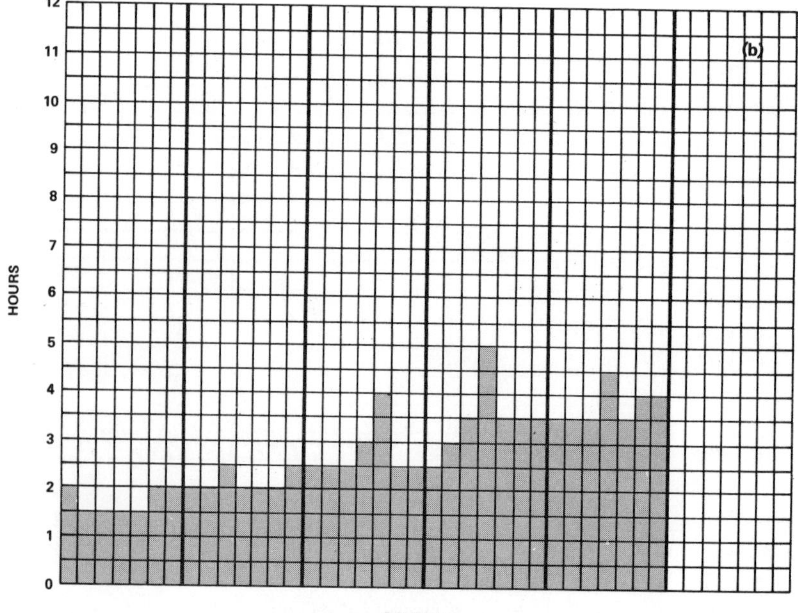

Fig. 26. Patient's graphs of (a) daily pain levels, and (b) daily time spent in goal-related activity.

chronic pain patients markedly decreased their pain levels and analgesic intakes, while greatly increasing their daily activities, and these improvements were sustained on follow-up after discharge from the hospital.

An important feature of the operant approach is the record keeping. Patients keep a daily log of their activities, accounting for every hour of the day (see Fig. 25), and record their average pain estimates for the day. Each day they draw graphs, abstracted from these logs, to mark their progress (see Fig. 26). As these are kept at their bedside, it gives the staff an opportunity to note and reinforce the patients' progress, and the patients too are able to see if they are attempting too much too fast, or are too cautious—in other words, they learn to acquire some cognitive control over acts which previously had been automatic. In addition, after a few weeks of such progress, patients are engaged in nearly a full day's work on goal-related activities, and gradually change their self-concepts. It is difficult to think of oneself as a chronic invalid when being active all day. The patients see—and it is displayed for the entire ward to observe—that they are capable of significant function in spite of their pain.

GROUP THERAPY

Although Fordyce *et al.* (26) have shown that the operant conditioning program is sufficient to rehabilitate pain patients, we have found it helpful to add group-treatment sessions. These are held daily for an hour, and are attended by all the pain patients, nurses on duty on the pain unit, and the psychologist. On one occasion per week, the surgeon attends also.

The purpose of these sessions is to give the patients an opportunity to express their concerns, to receive feedback from the staff and other patients about their behavior, and to learn some of the elementary principles of pain psychology as we have described them in this book—facts about depression, hypochondriasis, and pain games. The group sessions thus alternate between being like classes and like more traditional groups in psychiatric settings.

One of the benefits of these sessions is that the patients quickly realize that they are not alone, that others have been struggling and suffering and manipulating as they have, and that there is understanding of what they have been through. This seems to make for an *esprit de corps* which provides a setting in which patients feel more comfortable asking whether, for example, their low-back pain will lead to paralysis, or if they have cancer, and similar fears which they previously felt too inhibited to express.

This group support also makes less difficult the ability of patients to become aware of how they use their pain to receive payoffs such as sympathy, narcotics, financial compensation, or admiration for bravery. Such payoffs are usually not consciously conceived by the patients, and when this is presented in didactic fashion, the group tends to rally and protest their good intentions. However, once an individual patient has his pain game described to him by other patients who have had similar games, he is more inclined to accept it and analyze his behavior. This is more effective than when feedback is provided by the staff. Patients may deceive themselves and the staff, but they cannot long deceive the other patients with whom they are living, and feedback from the others, given supportively, soon stops the game playing.

Thus one of the chief functions of the therapy group is to expose, by making explicit, the misuse of pain as a weapon of interpersonal control, or as a means of persuading a doctor to do what the patient thinks ought to be done, or as any of the other kinds of payoffs which may make pain too important for a patient to give up even after an organic lesion has been corrected, thus preventing his rehabilitation.

Patients have felt so strongly about this aspect of the group that they continue these discussions among themselves on the ward, they have asked to have their spouses attend the sessions (which is permitted one day per week), and they frequently return after discharge, on the days of their outpatient follow-up visits.

Equally valued by the patients are the group meetings attended by the surgeons. Here, all the patients hear the surgeon report to individual patients the results of various diagnostic procedures, such as nerve conduction studies, nerve blocks, etc. Not only does the surgeon report the findings, but he analyzes the results and summarizes his thinking about the diagnostic and therapeutic possibilities. If he is unenthusiastic about trying a surgical procedure he says so, and gives his reasons. He may say, "Mr. Smith, before we did those spinal blocks, I was pretty sure your problem was at L4, rather than L5, and I still think so. But I'm reluctant to proceed any further, because you responded positively to a placebo block. By that I mean that you got as much pain relief from a shot of plain water as you did from the active blocking agent. Now that can mean a lot of things, such as the power of wishful thinking, or your trying to convince me to operate on you, but one thing I get from this is that you are not an accurate reporter of your pain, and I am not easily persuaded to undertake such a serious procedure on someone who does not report his symptoms accurately. What do you think?"

Similarly, the surgeon may tell Mr. Jones why he has not yet ordered certain tests for him. "You've been here as long as Mr. Smith, and seem to have a similar problem, but frankly speaking, as a surgeon, I simply don't know what to believe about what you say. Your complaint of suffering is so dramatic, your limp is so theatrical, that I would write you off completely if we didn't have some positive findings to go on. You've improved somewhat since you've been here, but I'm not yet convinced that you have a significant pain problem, and you're going to have to work harder with the staff here on what your difficulties really are. What have you learned since you've been here?"

And the surgeon may say to Mr. Brown, "We are sure now that your pain is causalgia, and it will respond to a sympathectomy. Do you want to have this performed, or can you live with your pain?" If Mr. Brown says he wants the operation, the surgeon may chide him for not asking about the risks first, and then go on to explain the temporary and permanent effects it will have. He will then insist that the patient think about it for several days, talk to his family, the staff, and the other patients, and then make up his mind (30).

Such sessions are very instructive to all the patients. It brings home to them the seriousness and the uncertainties of diagnostic and surgical procedures, so that they begin to perceive them as problem-solving efforts rather than some magical ritual. They see first hand the effect of their psychological processes on their symptoms, and how that affects the surgeon's reactions to them. And they learn, most importantly, how to communicate with physicians and surgeons, that is, what doctors look for in them, and how they must "read" the doctor. For patients who have made the rounds of clinics, doctors, and hospitals, becoming confused, frustrated, and bitter while earning every conceivable diagnostic label, this is a very enlightening process.

In these sessions, patients learn, for example, that if they insist on pain relief from a physician, then that physician can only provide analgesics. If they insist on relief from a surgeon, the surgeon's only recourse is an operative procedure. This apparently is not realized by most patients, who somehow have expected that "Mommy will kiss it and make it better." They learn, in other words, that if they have become addicted to narcotics, or have had unsuccessful or unnecessary surgery, then they had a lot to do with it; they are not passive recipients of medical actions.

It has become apparent to us that one of the most critical points in the treatment program is the explanation to the patient, by the surgeon, of the patient's physical *and* psychological status, and the feasibility of surgery. Until this point is reached, and the reasons for or against surgery are discussed by the surgeon, patients go through the proper motions of participating in the program but have obvious reservations about the psychological approach. They seem to be interested in showing how much they need surgery, and convey the impression that no real change in their life is needed as they may soon expect to be made whole again. Until the decision is made, only the surgeon carries enough credibility or influence with the patient to force a confrontation of the emotional factors in chronic pain. Once the decision about surgery is made, the program becomes more meaningful. Either surgery will not be done, in which case they must learn to live with their pain and make the best of it; or they will have surgery, and they can give up their reservations and get to work on their psychological problems.

The group-therapy sessions are also the setting in which resistance to treatment can be handled (since only positive reinforcement for progress is given on the ward.) It is an advantage of having specific behavioral goals, and of having daily charts on display at the bedside, that objective signs of improvement become important. What the patient intends, or what he says, is less important. Thus, although the patient may say he wants to spend increasing amounts of time learning shop work, if he actually fails to do so, then he evidences resistance.

This is brought out in group meetings, and the reasons for it discussed. The patient usually protests his good intentions, but we insist that "actions speak louder than words," and that if he does not do what he says he wants to do and agreed to do, then he is fooling us and himself, and it is senseless for him to remain in the program.

Another form of resistance takes the form of the patient's desire to talk about his physical condition. Many pain patients, in fact, show their only animation and enthusiasm when describing their symptoms or what the doctors have done to them in the past. When a patient does this, we, of course, point this out to him, showing him how he has focused all his interests and energy on his complaints, and noting that it will be difficult for him to give up this satisfaction. We insist, however, that we will have to interrupt such descriptions, first, because we find it boring, second because he needs to learn to get his satisfactions in other ways, and third, because such discussions prevent us from working at his and others' goals. Thereafter, we always interrupt such talk when it occurs.

Ultimately, most patients in our program make some improvement and are discharged. For those who do not receive surgery (it is not feasible, or it is declined), the average length of stay is about 6 weeks; it is somewhat longer for those receiving surgery, counting convalescent and physical rehabilitation periods. At the end of their stay we have a little ceremony for public recognition of their improvement, and award them a certificate (Fig. 27a). Occasionally a patient who plays the Confounder's game will not have benefited from his stay at all; he also will have earned a certificate of achievement (Fig. 27b).

EVALUATION OF THE TREATMENT PROGRAM

Probably no new program should be developed without a system for assessing its effectiveness. It is too easy for the therapists to be blinded by their enthusiasm for the enterprise, so that they are not properly critical or objective, and they and the patients can engage in mutual deception to reinforce each others' expectations. Therefore, every treatment program should have a built-in evaluation system, preferably with as objective data as possible, and these should be used to improve the program continually and to provide for critical inspection by others.

PAIN TREATMENT PROGRAM

This is to certify that

____

is a

* **PAIN EXPERT** *

who has learned to live well despite having pain, and so is entitled to the greatest admiration and respect.

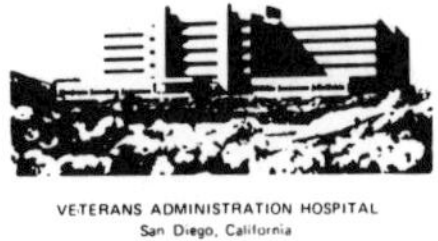

VETERANS ADMINISTRATION HOSPITAL
San Diego, California

____
Richard A. Sternbach, Ph.D.
Director

____
Date

(a)

PAIN TREATMENT PROGRAM

This is to certify that

____

is a

* **PERPETUAL PAIN PATIENT** *

who has defeated the best efforts of our specialists, and is to be congratulated for this achievement.

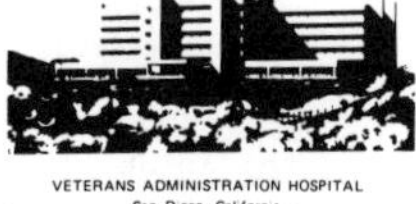

VETERANS ADMINISTRATION HOSPITAL
San Diego, California

____
Richard A. Sternbach, Ph.D.
Director

____
Date

(b)

Fig. 27. "Diplomas" awarded patients who complete the treatment program. (a) For those who have shown substantial improvement. (b) For some of those who have failed to benefit.

This should be easy to do with the kinds of data collection we have already described. The method of patient logs was first developed by Fordyce *et al.* (25), to whom we are indebted for this system, and we have already presented some of our results in Chapter VIII.

Of course, treatment programs will be particularized for individual patients, who will have different goals, different problems, and different criteria for success. For example, patients with postherpetic neuralgia of the arm, or pain from a brachial plexus avulsion, will probably not have any trouble walking, so that this will not be as useful a measure of change as it would be for those with low-back pain and sciatica. But, in general, activity levels of pain patients tend to be low, and increase with reduction of pain, and so changes in the amount and duration of activity can be an indirect measure of success.

Somewhat more specific is the amount of time spent on goal-related activities, whether this be working in a machine shop, studying for a new career, or indulging in a neglected hobby. To the extent that patients spend time in such activities they may be considered to be in a non-pain state, although this is not strictly true of course, they at least are engaging in activity which is rewarding, thus antithetical to suffering, and so a useful measure of improvement.

Another criterion which is sometimes cited is the decrease in analgesics used. This is difficult to measure when patients enter on a wide variety of medications, although Fordyce *et al.* (26) have used a method of converting analgesic intake into a proportion of a standard potent analgesic dosage. Certainly this is an important indirect measure of the success of a treatment program, for presumably analgesics requested and received reflect the patients' pain experience. This is not quite true in an inpatient program where medications are regulated and systematically decreased, for decreases then reflect more about the consistency of the administration of the program than changes in patients' pain experiences. Such a measure is more useful when the patients have returned home and can have readier access to analgesics. For this reason we have not measured the systematic decreases in analgesic intake during the treatment program, but have calculated pretreatment and follow-up equivalents.

Some investigators have argued that the only "hard" criterion of successful pain relief is the patients' return to work. While this is certainly an index of success, it is really too stringent an application of the work ethic, for some patients (e.g., poststroke anesthesia dolorosa) will remain too disabled to work despite pain relief. Others may have already retired prior to the onset of their pain, and still others may never have worked and have no need to. Activity—productive, useful, or rewarding—may be a good index, but work in the sense of gainful employment is not.

Another possible indirect measure of successful treatment is the objective personality test whose neurotic scales, as we have shown, are associated with pain complaints. If a treatment program is successful, such scales will show a change towards the normal range of scores. Such a change will be correlated not with any necessary decrease in pain levels, but with a changed outlook. The patients will either feel differently about themselves and the world because they have had significant pain relief, or they may be able to tolerate their pain better because their attitudes have changed. In any event, the changed scores should correlate with progress in treatment.

The most direct measures, of course, are those of the pain experience itself. The whole point of a pain treatment program is to abolish or significantly reduce the pain, whether by surgery, nonaddicting psychotropic medications, operant conditioning, or whatever, and all other measures of activities are really measures of the means by which this ultimate goal is achieved. It is the patients' description of their pain which, after all, causes them to be evaluated for treatment, and only some expression of a change in their pain experience can be used to assess the effectiveness of treatment. Therefore, the pain estimates made by the patients each day, and the tourniquet pain scores taken weekly, are most important, as shown in the previous chapter.

In Fig. 28 are shown the various pain and activity measures we have used, for all patients who completed the treatment program at the time of this writing. Figures 29 and 30 show the same measure for those patients who received

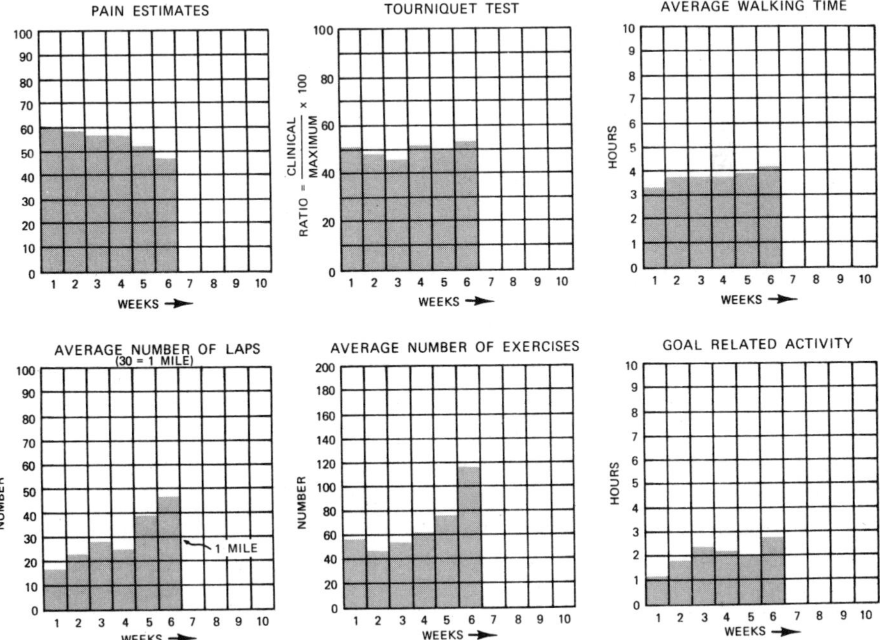

Fig. 28. Weekly changes in pain and activity levels for all patients in program $N = 75$.

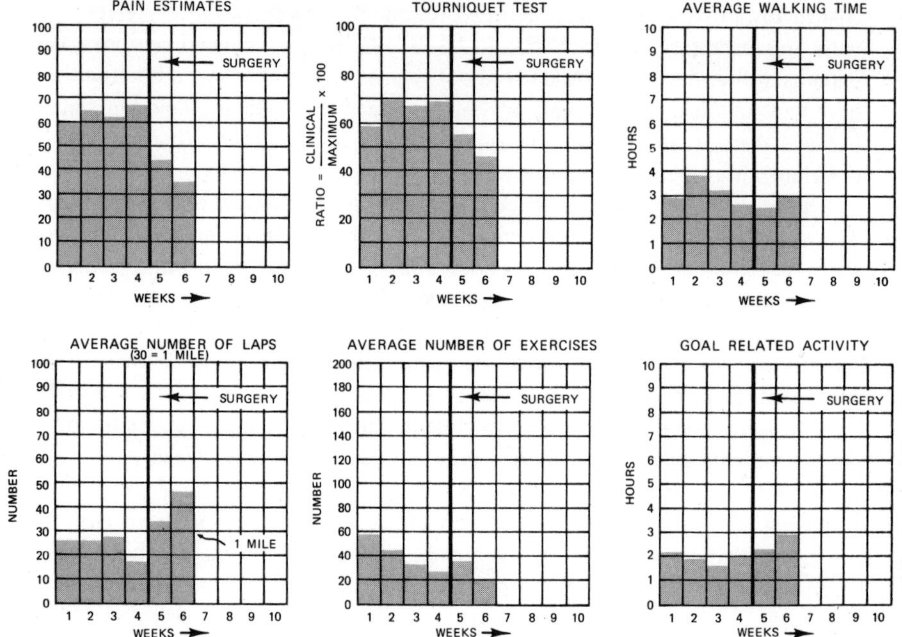

Fig. 29. Weekly changes in pain and activity levels for subgroup of patients who received surgical treatment for relief of pain, as well as psychological rehabilitation program, $N = 25$.

surgical treatment for their pain and those who did not, respectively. These illustrations show that pain levels, in general, fall—most dramatically with surgery—and activity levels increase. However, with those who do not receive surgical relief of their pain, pain levels increase in proportion to increased activity.

Pre- and posttreatment psychological test scores are shown for the total group of patients in Fig. 31. These profiles show significant improvement in Hypochondriasis, Depression, Hysteria, and Psychasthenia (anxiety). The two subgroups' profiles are shown in Figs. 32 and 33, and similar improvement (although not all significant) can be seen as for the total group.

It should be noted that for all the above measures, improvement is not a function of increased analgesics, but occurred despite systematic decreases in analgesic doses. Except for the subgroup of patients (about $\frac{1}{3}$ of the total) who experienced a dramatic decrease in pain with surgery, patients, in general, showed improvement in activity and outlook despite an increase in pain associated with their activities and decreased analgesic intake. An important

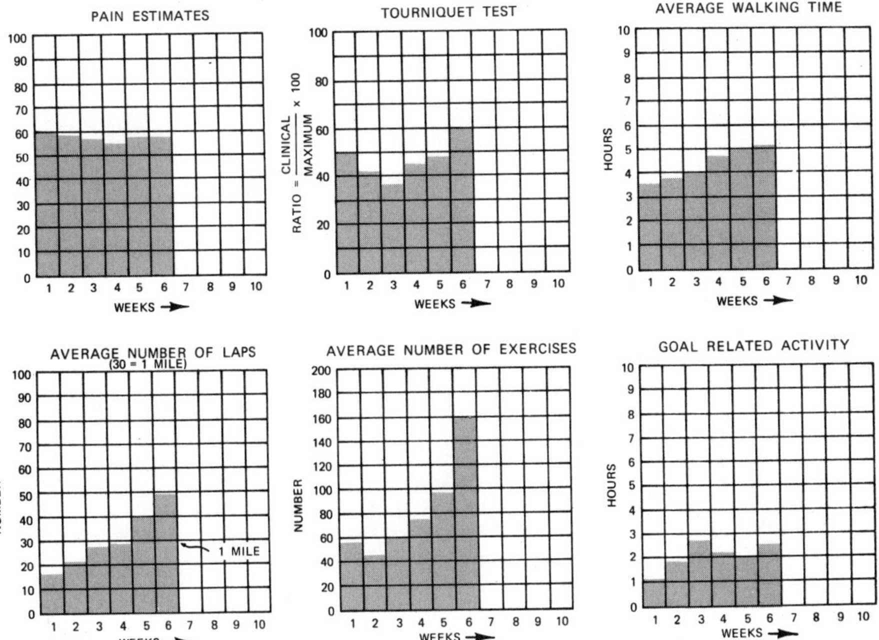

Fig. 30. Weekly changes in pain and activity levels for subgroup of patients who received psychological treatment only, $N = 50$.

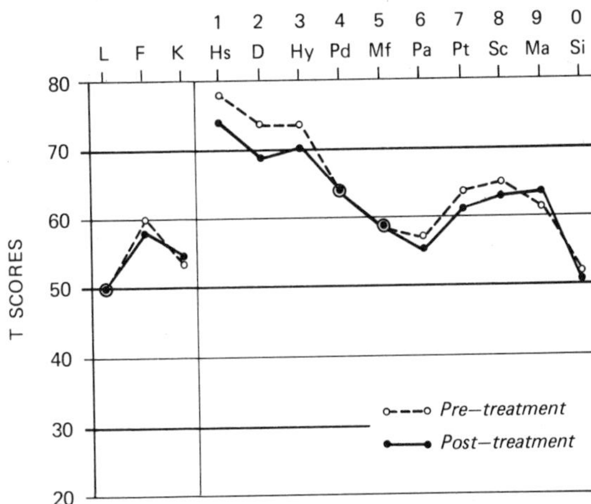

Fig. 31. MMPI profiles for total group, $N = 75$, before and after treatment. Differences on scales 1, 2, and 3 are significant.

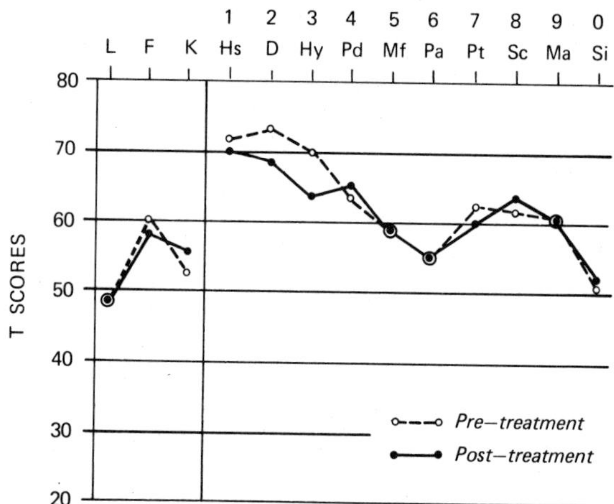

Fig. 32. MMPI profiles for patients who received surgery, $N = 25$, before and after treatment. A significant difference appears on scale 3.

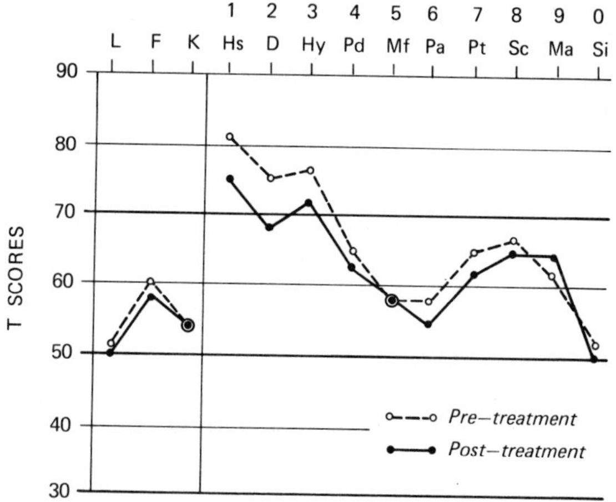

Fig. 33. MMPI profiles for patients who did not receive surgery, $N = 50$, before and after treatment. Significant differences appear on scales 1, 2, and 3.

question, then, is whether such improvements are maintained after discharge from the program. Follow-up information is critical in assessing the effectiveness of a treatment program in order to rule out transient nonspecific treatment effects.

Figure 34 shows the results of a 6-month follow-up on all patients from whom we were able to obtain data. These data show that improvement is maintained. The pain estimates can be compared with those shown in

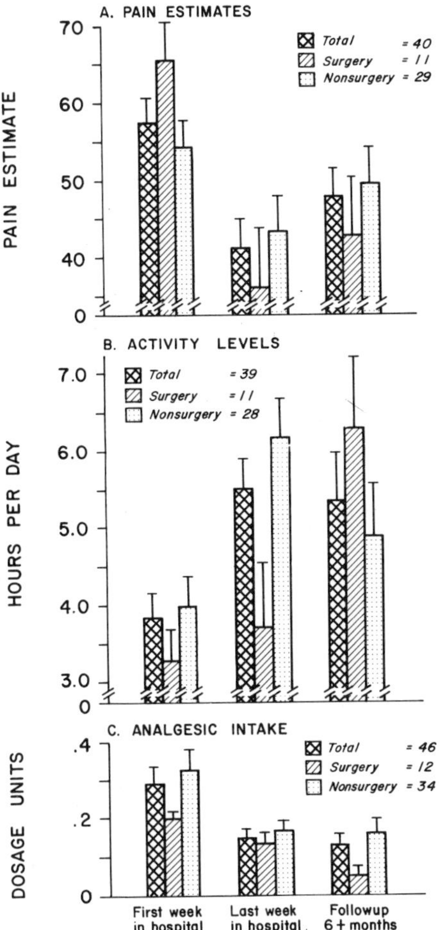

Fig. 34. Follow-up data on patients discharged 6 mo or longer; 61 questionnaires mailed, 67% returned. Averages shown are comparable to those of the larger group on first and last weeks of hospital stay. (A) Pain estimates, means and standard errors shown. Significant decreases occur between the first and last weeks in the hospital for the total group ($p < 0.001$) and for the surgery ($p < 0.05$) and nonsurgery ($p < 0.001$) subgroups. On follow-up, the total group still has significantly less pain ($p < 0.05$) than on admission, as does the surgery subgroup ($p < 0.02$), but the nonsurgery subgroup's estimates are no longer significantly lower. (B) Activity levels, showing means and standard errors of the number of hours per day in worklike activity (not resting). The difference between the first and last weeks in the hospital is significant for the total group ($p < 0.001$) and for the nonsurgery subgroup ($p < 0.001$), but is not for the surgery subgroup (still recovering from surgery). On follow-up, the levels remain significantly increased from admission for the total

Figs. 28–30, and it will be seen that they continue to show a lessened pain experience despite a continued lower analgesic intake and sustained increases in activity.

ADDITIONAL TREATMENT METHODS

We have thus far described these major treatment approaches for chronic pain patients: operant conditioning, group therapy in the ward milieu, and antidepressants as indicated. These are general approaches that are of value to most patients, and are directed to the patients' rehabilitation. The general methods, of course, are tailored to the individual patients' choice of a more desirable future life-style.

Apart from the three major techniques, there are some additional ones which are not useful for all patients, but do benefit some. These are methods which are more specifically aimed at providing symptomatic relief, i.e., the temporary reduction or abolition of pain.

Sensory Stimulation

Since the proposal of a new, gate control theory of pain by Melzack and Wall (48), there has been a resurgence of interest in what was formerly called the "counter-irritant" method of pain control. It has long been known, on an empirical basis, that vigorous stimulation of any sensory modality will cause a marked decrease or disappearance of pain for varying periods of time. Since such stimulation is "natural" and usually quite benign, treatment by this method is preferable to destructive surgery or addicting medications, and so it is understandable that with the rationale of the gate-control theory behind them, some investigators are now exploring this approach more systematically.

The gate-control theory of pain predicts that stimulation of larger diameter sensory fibers will excite gating cells in the substantia gelatinosa, inhibiting the transmission of impulses from smaller fibers responding to noxious or pain stimuli (48). Several studies lend support to this view. Melzack and Schecter (47) reported that itch intensity was reduced by vibration applied either to the stimulated or to the contralateral area. Wall and Sweet (88) reported that

---

group ($p < 0.05$) and for the surgery subgroup ($p < 0.01$), but the nonsurgery subgroup's activity is no longer significantly greater. (C) Analgesic intake, expressed in dosage units calculated as a proportion of the strength of an effective dose of morphine (26). The decreases from the first to the last week of hospitalization are significant for the total group ($p < 0.01$), and for the surgery ($p < 0.02$) and the nonsurgery ($p < 0.01$) subgroups. On follow-up, the decrease is still significantly different than the first week of admission for the total group ($p < 0.01$), and for the surgery ($p < 0.001$) and the nonsurgery ($p < 0.05$) subgroups.

in patients with chronic severe cutaneous pain, 2 minutes of electrical stimulation of the sensory nerves or roots resulted in temporary abolition of the pain, in some cases outlasting the stimulation by more than half an hour.

Sullivan (81) was able to increase the lower pain threshold to radiant heat by vibrating the area, the degree of increase being correlated with the frequency of vibrations. Higgins *et al.* (33) found that the ipsilateral application of a dynamic tactile stimulus, an inflating cuff, significantly raised the upper threshold to cutaneous electric shock. Satran and Goldstein (65) reported that cutaneous electrical stimulation increased the maximum tolerance for pain due to electrical shock, and furthermore that it suppressed the somatosensory cortical evoked potential.

These studies support the gate-control prediction, that larger fiber stimulation inhibits the transmission cephalad of pain impulses, the inhibition presumably occurring at the level of the spinal cord. Accordingly, it is reasonable to suppose that for certain patients, whose pain is localized and appropriate to an understandable lesion, the application of a vibrator, or a transcutaneous electrical neural stimulator, may provide relief.

Melzack (personal communication, 1972) has reported success in a few cases of tic douloreaux, using a vibrator for about 10 minutes, four or five times daily. The patient begins to massage at the periphery of the painful area, and gradually, over a period of days, approaches the trigger point. In a few weeks the patients are free of pain. In our own experience, which is haphazard, central pain states seem to be worsened with such stimulation, two cases of anesthesia dolorosa and two of postherpetic neuralgia being particularly refractory. On the other hand, patients with peripheral nerve injuries occasionally report gratifying relief. This has been particularly true of several patients with headaches following neck trauma and cervical fusions, and some low-back and sciatica patients. The latter, particularly, seem to benefit from transcutaneous neural stimulators, unless there has been a fusion or excessive scarring on the sensory roots.

An interesting phenomenon is that with electrical stimulation, when it provides relief, patients report that after a time they require stimulation for shorter periods, and the intervals between stimulation periods can be lengthened. This suggests that some tonic activation of the pain inhibitory gate may be occurring, and this hypothesis deserves systematic investigation.

Biofeedback

Testing the hypothesis that the α state is incompatible with being in severe pain (which normally produces activation), Gannon and Sternbach (28) reported on a case with postconcussion headaches who underwent α training. In time, the patient was able to avoid headaches by inducing α, but could not end the headaches by this means.

Since then we have used α training on a number of patients whose pain levels seemed associated with levels of tension or activation, and all reported good reduction in pain levels. Much more effective, however, is the muscle or electromyogram feedback. Budzynski *et al.* (13) reported on the effectiveness of this method for the treatment of tension headaches. We have found this very efficient, requiring only four or five sessions of half an hour in length before the patient reports significant relief. Similarly, muscle spasms respond very favorably, patients soon learning to acquire control of the affected muscle groups and to prevent the cramping. Two cases of spasmodic torticollis failed to correct their head turning, but did learn muscle relaxation and thus diminished the associated pain.

These are uncontrolled observations, taking place in the setting of the total treatment program previously described, and with all the effects of suggestion, role playing, etc., contaminating the results. However, there is an extensive research literature of biofeedback methods, in which appropriate controls are employed, and this need not concern us here. Those interested in teaching patients methods of pain control will find that α or muscle biofeedback training is quite effective for appropriate patients.

Hypnosis

There is an enormous literature on hypnosis, and a goodly amount of it pertains to the relief of pain states. All the papers on the subject, of course, recommend it, some giving illustrative case histories, most simply talking about the procedure in general terms, but none of the reports I have been able to find are worth citing. There are no quantitative data nor follow-up results, and there is little to recommend them except for the general consensus that hypnosis can provide pain relief in many instances.

Were I a devotee of the method I would use it more extensively, for whatever works to reduce pain and is so benign is worth trying. In our program, we teach self-hypnosis to help patients go to sleep at night, for many patients report that when they can keep busy during the day their pain does not bother them, however, the pain seems much worse when other stimuli are reduced while they are trying to fall asleep. Accordingly, if there are several such patients in the program, or if an "epidemic" of insomnia sweeps the ward (which occasionally happens), then one of the group sessions is given over to instructions in self-hypnosis, involving a focus of attention on slow, deep breathing, muscle relaxation, etc. Approximately $\frac{1}{3}$ of the patients take the trouble to practice the technique, and most of them find it very effective for getting to sleep with no intrusion from their pain.

We make no special claims for hypnosis as a pain reliever, and keep no separate records which would permit its evaluation. We mention the technique simply because it has an ancient history for this purpose, it is rather harmless, and although not all patients can be (or want to be) hypnotized, some can, and the method will undoubtedly help them control or "rise above" their pain.

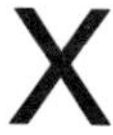

Special Issues

The following topics are among those which have been asked about by professionals who have considered establishing a pain clinic or treatment program.

"FIRST, DO NO HARM"

Those who practice the healing professions usually follow certain principles, and foremost is the injunction to "heal the sick, and comfort the suffering." Patients with chronic benign pain are certainly among the suffering, and those who examine and treat such patients are very liable to do all in their power to heal the disease causing the pain, or failing that, to diminish the suffering.

Unfortunately, the principles of compassion, concern, and care which are appropriate to acute pain patients do not seem to benefit patients with long-lasting pain, and indeed there comes a time during the transition from acute to chronic status when the most helpful information the healer can give the patient is that the pain condition is not likely to change, that it will have to be endured, and the patient will have to give thought to how he wishes to live the rest of his life in spite of the pain.

It comes as a surprise to many doctors and nurses to learn that "TLC" (Tender, Loving Care) actually undermines the patient's efforts at rehabilitation. Such sympathetic attention cannot easily be put aside by the patient who likes it, nor by the staff for whom it is the only response in the repertoire. But whereas "TLC" is indeed healing in acute injury or disease states, it prolongs indefinitely the sick role. Once the condition has stabilized, and pain becomes chronic, "Poor dear!" must give way to "You're feeling sorry for yourself," if the patient makes no effort to take up his life again. Similarly, analgesics which are such a blessing in the acute phase apparently become exacerbating in the chronic phase.

In this connection, the role of the doctor must be considered. If a patient complains of pain, the doctor must attempt to discover the cause. Suppose no cause or a benign noncorrectible condition is found. Is the doctor to relieve the pain anyway? If so, how?

As one who has seen very many pain patients who have been to many clinics and hospitals, I have had the opportunity to observe how much harm has been done by well-intentioned doctors who have tried to "comfort the suffering." I have myself, early on, collaborated in the decision to perform the fifty-fifth surgical procedure on a patient with phantom limb pain, a procedure which turned out to be as valueless as the preceding fifty-four. I have seen patients, with totally negative findings on all physical diagnostic tests, so thoroughly addicted to potent narcotics that government agents were investigating the doctors, pharmacists, and patients involved. Clearly, there must be some corollary principle to "comfort the suffering" which will prevent such absurdities.

I suggest that one possible modifier of that dictum is a division of responsibility between doctor and patient. The doctor does not have the responsibility to treat pain, or rather to silence the complaint of pain but rather a responsibility to detect and treat pathology. The patient, on the other hand, has the responsibility of providing organic pathology in order to justify treatment; his complaint of pain does not by itself justify the prescription of strong analgesics or surgical intervention, no matter how apparent his suffering seems.

This is rather a radical suggestion. It might seem as though I am suggesting that doctors ignore pain, which is not the case at all. What I am suggesting is that doctors should identify the pathology causing the pain symptom, and unless they are quite sure about what that is, they should be very hesitant in their intervention. An example can illustrate this point.

CASE ILLUSTRATION 10

Mr. G. F. is a 77-year-old man who was referred by an oncologist because of complaints of persistent severe pain in the left temporo-mandibular area, varying in primary location from the tongue to the ear.

This pain began about $2\frac{1}{2}$ years ago following the surgical removal of radium needles placed following excision of a malignancy of the tongue. Although there is no evidence of recurrence of the malignancy, the pain has persisted, and is described by the patient as "excruciating."

In the spring of this year, Mr. F.—by his own admission—talked a neurosurgeon into sectioning branches of the Vth and IXth nerves, and has had three stellate ganglion blocks. None of these has provided permanent relief. Mr. F. takes one Percodan every 3 hours while awake, with whiskey, and one Nembutal at bedtime, plus another if awakened during the night.

Interview and Recent History. Mr. F. is accompanied by his wife, who is 74. Both look much younger than their ages. He has some left-sided weakness and numbness, a consequence of his surgical procedures, walks awkwardly with a cane, and drools from the left corner of his mouth. Mrs. F. notes that the last surgery "took a lot out of him. He's not like he was."

They have been married $1\frac{1}{2}$ years, both having been widowed just a short time earlier. Mr. F. had no children, but Mrs. F. has a daughter and three grandchildren living nearby. Mr. F. retired 16 years ago, and on his savings and retirement income they take extensive trips around the world. He used to enjoy hunting and fishing a great deal, but cannot do that any more. When not traveling, he enjoys reading and watching TV. He says (and his wife confirms) that he is never bored, and although he drinks a great deal of whiskey every day, that has been his habit all his adult life. In the interview he joked, teased, and seemed in good spirits. There was no sign of distress or suffering, although the patient insisted he had to get rid of the pain, and noted that he had spent $15,000 on surgery and medicines, was left partly paralyzed, and still had the pain.

Test Findings. Mr. F. estimates the usual severity of his pain, on the 0–100 scale, as 75. This is a severe pain rating. However, on the tourniquet pain test, his clinical pain intensity was matched at 1 min 15 sec, and his maximum pain tolerance was reached in 3 min 55 sec. Thus his usual clinical pain is 32% of his tolerance. This is in the slight to moderate range, and far less than the severe 75% he estimated.

On the Health Index, there was no significant endorsement of items relating to chronic invalidism, manifest depression, or problems with doctors; however, there was a moderate amount of pain preoccupation.

The MMPI shows a significant potential for physical complaints (Fig. 35). He shows a mild to moderate depressive reaction which is masked to some extent by a tendency to deny emotional upsets or worries. The depression may possibly be a response to the pain, but it is equally probable that the pain is a consequence of the depression. This is particularly likely in view of the dramatic way he describes the pain, and his contradictory appearance of good spirits, suggestive of *la belle indifference* in conversion reactions. The test profile also indicates some unusual thought processes, indicative of a certain amount of confusion, daydreaming, and disorientation which often characterizes schizoid persons who present vague physical complaints rather than overt psychotic signs. Thus, it is likely that Mr. F.'s experience of physical pain is serving to mask the pain due to feelings of lowered efficiency and self-esteem.

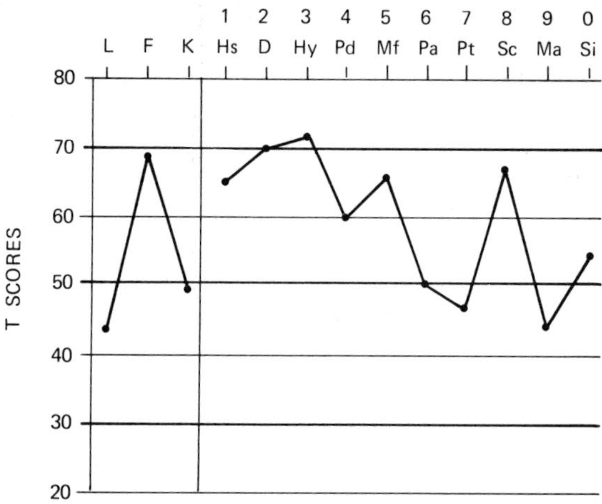

Fig. 35. MMPI profile of patient G. F.

Diagnostic Impression. Hysterical neurosis, conversion type (300.13), with depressive and schizoid features.

Recommendations. If Mr. F.'s liver function tests are adequate, a precaution necessary because of his age and drinking history, he would be a good candidate for the combination of amitriptyline and fluphenazine, which is often of benefit in chronic organic pain states which are potentiated by such psychological problems as his. However, dosages would have to be small to begin with, as Mr. F. is not likely to change his drinking habits. Furthermore, there seems to be no justification at this point for continuing the narcotics, as Mr. F. does not have severe pain, and discontinuance would be necessary to avoid the depressive effects of drug interactions.

PSYCHIATRIC CONSULTATIONS

Most psychiatrists seldom have the opportunity to deal with chronic pain patients in treatment, and so it is understandable that they may miss the nuances of personality which we discuss in this book when it comes to making a diagnosis. As compared with the typical psychiatric outpatient, the pain patient seems superficially not to be disturbed. In the clinical interview and mental status examination, there is rarely any sign of disorientation or thought disorder. Affect usually seems appropriate, and if there is any sign of depression, anxiety, or agitation, it usually seems rather mild and in proportion to the physical disability and discomfort.

Consequently, psychiatrists are understandably reluctant to prescribe psychotropic medications. The common feeling is that the patients do not seem to require them, or that the effective dose is so small (compared to that required for psychiatric patients) as to be "homeopathic" or possibly a "placebo."

What is overlooked, in this view, is that the depression that is present is usually masked, that it and the hypochondriasis and invalid life-style continually reinforce each other, and that there is little chance of breaking into this cycle and producing significant therapeutic gains without the aid of psychotropic medications.

Furthermore, there is increasing evidence that the tricyclic antidepressants and the phenothiazines have analgesic effects which are probably independent of changes they induce in mood and thinking. Recently, for example, Merskey and Hester (52) and Taub and Collins (85) have reported on their series of patients with chronic intractable pain due to nervous system lesions, who obtained good relief of pain from combinations of antidepressants and phenothiazines and, in some instances, antihistamines (52). Our own experience supports their findings, i.e., doses of amitriptyline as low as 75–100 mg q.h.s. often makes chronic pain quite bearable, and when the pain is severe, the addition of fluphenazine 2.5–5.0 mg q.d. seems to effect a significant improvement, so that small doses of non-narcotic analgesics (salicylates) are often adequate.

These results suggest that psychiatrists should not need to see a full-blown psychiatric profile before prescribing psychotropic medications for the management of chronic pain patients. They also suggest that pain and its relief may be in part a function of the neurohumoral balance in the brain stem, in particular, the relative availability of the monoamines in the mesencephalic central gray area (1,2,44) or perhaps the relative proportion of serotonin or dopamine to norepinephrine.

THE ROLE OF ANXIETY

The relationship of anxiety and pain has been extensively studied, and the manipulation of anxiety in experimental pain research has been a favorite strategy. However, there has been much less work with anxiety in the setting where chronic clinical pain has been the subject of inquiry. The reason seems to be that anxiety plays much less of a role in these conditions than does depression, whereas it is a major factor influencing pain in the acute state.

A classical example of the latter is the work by Egbert *et al.* (22), who found that the reduction of anxiety by preoperative instructions and encouragement, resulted in patients' postoperative narcotic requirements being halved, and in their being ready for discharge 2.7 days earlier, when compared with a control group who did not receive such treatment.

Similar work has been reported by Dalrymple *et al.* (20), who found in a study of 50 women having cholecystectomy, that those whose preoperative Neuroticism scores (on the Eysenck Personality Inventory) were high, tended to have greater postoperative pain and vital capacity impairment. These studies were repeated on 50 men who received surgery for peptic ulcers. Again, there were highly significant correlations between the Neuroticism score and postoperative pain, the number of narcotic injections required, and chest complications (55). Inasmuch as anxiety is a major component in this Neuroticism score, it is clear that the effect it has on the acute pain situation is quite dramatic.

Such nonspecific, generalized anxiety as may be reflected in a global neuroticism score seems less prominent in chronic pain states. With time, anxious concerns seem to become focused and to emerge as hypochondriasis, while the anxious affect and mood are replaced by a depressed affect and mood.

This is not to say that anxiety, as a clinical feature, is not present in chronic pain patients. It is indeed, and we may recall that a sizeable minority in Merskey's and Spear's (53) series carried a diagnosis of anxiety hysteria (anxiety neurosis, we should say.) However, despite the diagnoses, anxiety as a feature seems less prominent than depression. In support of this, although it can be considered circular reasoning, we may note that chronic pain patients seldom benefit from such proven antianxiety agents as chlordiazepoxide or diazepam, whereas they usually respond favorably to the tricyclic antidepressants at dosages which are quite unpleasant to normals. Yet the antidepressant which seems to have the best result, as judged from trial–and–error experience at several centers, is amitriptyline, which also has a sedative or antianxiety effect (52,74,85).

Such reasoning, i.e., inferring a diagnosis from the response to treatment, is of course suspect, but we have already made the case for the prominence of depression on other grounds, and merely cite these observations as additional evidence. Anxiety is usually the dominant feature when we visit the dentist, are injured, or acutely ill, or undergoing surgery, but it has clearly been overplayed in experimental pain research. If an equivalent amount of effort were given to research on chronic pain and depression, we would be much further along in treating chronic pain patients.

OUTPATIENT TREATMENT?

It is obviously very expensive to work up and treat patients in the manner described in the previous chapter, and in view of the time, expense, and great number of such patients, it would be preferable to be able to do this on an outpatient basis. Would this be possible or effective?

Prior to initiating the inpatient Pain Unit, the author had run three groups of chronic pain patients as outpatients for 1 year. In one, the co-therapist was a psychiatric resident; in one, a psychiatric social worker; and in one, a full-time faculty staff psychiatrist. Of the 24 patients, 20 were low-back pain patients. All 24 had been thoroughly worked up and had been told that no further surgery was possible to correct any defect (most had had several surgeries), nor was pain-relieving surgery feasible. All agreed to the group treatment ($1\frac{1}{2}$ hours per week) in order to learn better how to live with their pain. Of the 24, only 1 showed any improvement at the end of the year.

In relating these findings to the staff of our narcotics treatment program, as one of a series of seminars on faculty research interests, the staff members were much amused. It was they who first pointed out to me that what I had been dealing with was a certain kind of life-style, and they (the ex-addicts) knew a great deal about that. There was no chance of changing a life-style outside a therapeutic community, they said, and then they regaled me with stories of how they had complained of pain and, in some instances, submitted to surgery, in order to obtain prescription narcotics.

These people may have overstated their case, but it was true that the pain patients bore some resemblance to addicts and alcoholics in the persistence of their life-style and in the lack of impact obtained from outpatient therapy. Between sessions, the patients went to various private doctors, to clinics, and chiropractors, and spent much of their time during the sessions describing either these visits or their symptoms. We had no control over their reinforcers—family, friends, doctors, medications. We made no headway.

This was the rationale behind starting the inpatient unit, in which payoffs can be changed, and in which patients begin to change their behavior, or life-style, and have an opportunity to see the results. An inpatient setting provides a consistent milieu in which treatment can be effective. Without such a setting, it is unlikely that chronic pain patients can get better.

It should be recalled that a full 20% of Penman's (56) trigeminal neuralgia patients failed to recover despite satisfactory block of nerve. Similar results obtain in a variety of surgical procedures for pain relief, although the rates differ according to the nature of the pain generator and the surgery employed. I have no doubt that if a magical pill were developed tomorrow which "should" abolish pain, a very significant proportion of chronic pain patients would continue to complain of pain, and indeed "have" it by all objective criteria. This is because they have so altered their lives that they need the pain, and cannot live without it. Outpatient treatment would not make much of an impact on them. It is not difficult to understand then that outpatient treatment is not likely to help those who have both the somatic pain generator and the psychological problems too.

The only part of the program which seems to be applicable to an outpatient setting is that involving the collecting of data. It is reasonable to expect a fairly accurate keeping of activity levels and pain estimates and medication intakes, for patients consciously hope that such data will help the doctor make a new diagnosis which will result in some new treatment. Indeed, Fordyce (personal communication, 1971) has patients keep a 2-week log as part of the psychological assessment for the University of Washington Pain Clinic, which is only diagnostic in function.

It is well to keep diagnostic and treatment functions separate in one's thinking, unless it is administratively possible to merge them as described in the previous chapter. If this cannot be done, then most diagnostic procedures can probably be performed in the outpatient clinic, but treatment—whether surgical, or behavioral rehabilitation—will require the structure of the inpatient setting.

SELECTION OF PATIENTS

We have already (Chapter VIII) indicated that it is possible to predict, on psychological grounds, which patients will do well and which will do poorly in treatment, irrespective of the nature of the physical diagnosis. Such predictions can be made by any program which takes all applicants and develops its own criteria and statistics. At some point, it may be desirable to start screening out those whose problems are not likely to be amenable to the treatment program.

One of the most pressing issues is that raised by the surgeon, who wants to know of the psychologist whether or not a particular patient is a "safe" candidate for surgery, that is, not so disturbed as to claim pain after a procedure which "should" abolish it. I feel very strongly that if such surgery is feasible and warranted on neurological grounds, and the patient agrees, then it must never be withheld because of the patient's psychological profile. A totally psychotic patient can have a bad disc or causalgia, and he is as entitled to a laminectomy or sympathectomy as anyone else. To judge otherwise on psychiatric grounds alone is unethical discrimination, in my view, and a perversion of psychodiagnostic techniques.

However, I well understand the concern, both for the patient and for the surgeon; for the patient, that he not continue with his pain after the operation; and for the surgeon, that he not go through an extensive and serious procedure only to fail because the patient has emotional problems. The solution that we have developed, as indicated in the previous chapter, is that the surgeon and patient agree on what will be done, but the timing of it often depends on the patient's psychological progress—with the full understanding and agreement of the patient. We have had a few patients, after surgery was offered to them, who requested no further psychological treatment. They were promptly transferred and received their surgery. However, most patients, knowing that they could now expect neurosurgical intervention, were willing to spend another few weeks if necessary to ensure that their pain did not persist for such psychological reasons as drug addiction or altered family relationships.

An alternative approach is to separate the psychological and somatic programs altogether, so that in the psychological treatment program are only those patients who have no physical findings, and/or those for whom no more somatic therapies are possible. This division may save time and avoid contamination of one issue by another, but it has the drawback that it deprives patients of the therapeutic benefits of mixing with different kinds of patients. It is very instructive to both those who will receive surgery, and those who will not, to sit in a group and hear the reasons why.

At some point in the development of a treatment program, decisions must be made about whether patients will be included who have no physical findings, i.e., are diagnosed "psychogenic" by exclusion of other causes; whether terminal or malignant pain patients will be accepted; whether diagnosis and treatment will be made separate functions; and whether the psychological and somatic approaches will be performed sequentially or in parallel. In addition, some restriction may be made on the kind of physical diagnoses which will be treated. Will there be an emphasis on back patients? Will headache or arthritis patients be accepted?

Such considerations as these seem to be of greater importance than that of predicting and selecting the patients who will be well. They reflect the philosophy of the program, and that, in turn, will depend upon the administrative structure of the organization.

ADMINISTRATIVE CONCERNS

It is probably not possible to develop a diagnostic pain clinic, or a pain treatment program, if it is not the chief professional interest of the majority of the staff. If several persons get together to establish such a program because it seems like good public relations for their institution, or a financially profitable venture, then it will probably go badly for everyone. At least two persons should have pain as their major commitment: a psychologist or psychiatrist; and a neurosurgeon or anesthesiologist. Other participating specialists, such as orthopedists, physiatrists, and neurologists, should also be prepared to devote a substantial proportion of their time to this endeavour, and all parties should expect and want to learn a great deal about pain mechanisms and pain patients.

One professional will have to devote full time to the administration of the program. This involves teaching the nursing and rehabilitation staffs, supervising the collection and analysis of data, corresponding about referrals, making decisions about patient flow, coordinating conferences and consultations, and in general ensuring a high quality of patient care and record keeping. Without such an administrator it is likely that many details will be overlooked, staffing of patients will be disorganized, and many cases will "fall between the cracks," with resulting poor morale and ineffective treatment. If the administrator is a psychologist, one of the M.D.'s will have to be medical director of the program, and in any case each patient will have to have one physician who will be medically responsible for him.

Ground rules and role specifications should be carefully thought out and made explicit. The patients who will be seen are desperate and have great magical expectations, and in order to help them develop a realistic life-style, by means of frank and open communications, the staff must expect to set the pattern. This means, for example, that a clear distinction must be made between experimental procedures and established ones. What will be the staff attitude towards the colleague who is interested in implanting stimulating electrodes? What will be the reception of the colleague who is enthusiastic about his results with acupuncture? What about trials of a promising new analgesic or antidepressant? If such techniques are considered experimental, will the structure of the organization permit appropriate experimental controls, with patients giving truly full and informed consent with no coercion? Will there be frank discussions with all patients about why some are chosen to participate in the research and some are not? (The word will surely get out, and patients will want to know.) Will there be institutional review by a human experimentation committee? And finally, who will be responsible for making decisions about such issues?

Once a clinic or program gets established, two other phenomena are sure to develop. Trainees in various professional programs begin to appear, requesting participation as part of their career development. They wish to observe, or do research of some sort, occasionally seeking sponsorship from one of the staff. Their motivation is usually one of interest, pain being somewhat more fascinating than the traditional subject areas in the several disciplines it cuts across. Some decision will have to be made about the extent to which patients will be exploited for such purposes; patients are people, and do not like to be thought of as being in a zoo, and a stream of observers or researchers can disrupt treatment. Nevertheless, professional training is a legitimate function, and some can be permitted. A useful guide is that any participant–observer must be able to give something useful or therapeutic back to the patients, or else it is a one-way, exploiting relationship.

The second phenomenon which develops is the request for information by reporters from newspapers, magazines, and television. Similar considerations apply here. On the one side is the need for the program to communicate with potential patients and referring physicians, and the right of the public to know about the program. On the other side is the concern of the program not to offend other professionals, not to be misrepresented by distorted reporting, not to raise false hopes in patients, and not to permit an invasion of patients' privacy. A compromise lies in the screening of potential reporters by the reputation of their medium and the quality of their work.

Although such matters as these seem trivial, in fact they involve problems which do not go away by ignoring them, and unless they are dealt with properly they can have a deleterious effect on the diagnostic and therapeutic functions of a program. Thus, careful attention to administrative details is essential to the success of the program.

Bibliography

1. Akil, H. Monaminergic mechanisms underlying stimulation-produced analgesia. Doctoral dissertation, University of California, Los Angeles, 1972.
2. Akil, H., and Mayer, D. J. Antagonism of stimulation-produced analgesia by *p* CPA, a serotonin synthesis inhibitor. *Brain Research,* 1972, **44**, 692–697.
3. Baker, J. W., and Mersky, H. Pain in general practice. *Journal of Psychosomatic Research,* 1967, **10**, 383–387.
4. Battista, A. F., and Wolff, B. B. Levodopa and induced-pain response: A study of patients with parkinsonian and pain syndromes. *Archives of Internal Medicine,* 1973, **132**, 70–74.
5. Bender, B. Seven angry crocks. *Psychosomatics,* 1964, **5**, 225–229.
6. Berne, E. *Games People Play.* New York: Grove Press, 1964.
7. Berne, E. *What Do You Say After You Say Hello?: The Psychology of Human Destiny.* New York: Grove Press, 1971.
8. Bond, M. R. The relation of pain to the Eysenck Personality Inventory, Cornell Medical Index and Whiteley Index of Hypochondriasis. *British Journal of Psychiatry,* 1971, **119**, 671–678.
9. Bond, M. R., and Pearson, I. B. Psychological aspects of pain in women with advanced cancer of the cervix. *Journal of Psychosomatic Research,* 1969, **13**, 13–19.
10. Bond, M. R., and Pilowsky, I. Subjective assessment of pain and its relationship to the administration of analgesics in patients with advanced cancer. *Journal of Psychosomatic Research,* 1966, **10**, 203–208.
11. Bonime, W. The Psychodynamics of Neurotic Depression. In S. Arieti (Ed.), *American Handbook of Psychiatry,* Vol. 3. New York: Basic Books, 1966.
12. Bradley, J. J. Severe localized pain associated with the depressive syndrome. *British Journal of Psychiatry,* 1963, **109**, 741–745.
13. Budzynski, T., Stoyva, J., and Adler, C. Feedback-induced muscle relaxation: Application to tension headache. *Journal of Behavior Therapy and Experimental Psychiatry,* 1970, **1**, 205–211.
14. Cassidy, W. L., Flanagan, N. B., Spellman, B. A., and Cohen, M. E. Clinical observations in manic-depressive disease: A quantitative study of one hundred manic-

depressive patients and fifty medically sick controls. *Journal of the American Medical Association,* 1957, **164,** 1535–1546.

15. Castelnuovo-Tedesco, P., and Krout, B. M. Psychosomatic aspects of chronic pelvic pain. *International Journal of Psychiatry in Medicine,* 1970, **1,** 109–126.
16. Chrzanowski, G. Neurasthenia and hypochondriasis. In S. Arieti (Ed.), *American Handbook of Psychiatry,* Vol. I. New York: Basic Books, 1959.
17. Comrey, A. L. A factor analysis of items on the MMPI Hypochondriasis scale. *Educational and Psychological Measurement,* 1957, **17,** 568–577.
18. Comrey, A. L. A factor analysis of items on the MMPI Depression scale. *Educational and Psychological Measurement,* 1957, **17,** 578–585.
19. Dahlstrom, W. G., Welsh, G. S., and Dahlstrom, L. E., *An MMPI Handbook,* Vol. I. *Clinical Interpretation* (rev. ed.). Minneapolis, Minn: University of Minnesota Press, 1972.
20. Dalrymple, D. G., Parbrook, G. D., and Steel, D. F. The effect of personality on postoperative pain and vital capacity impairment. *British Journal of Anaesthesia,* 1972, **44,** 902.
21. Diamond, S. Depressive headaches. *Headache,* 1964, **4,** 255–258.
22. Egbert, L. D., Battit, G. E., Welch, C. E., and Bartlett, M. K. Reduction of postoperative pain by encouragement and instruction of patients. *New England Journal of Medicine,* 1964, **270,** 825–827.
23. Engel, G. L. "Psychogenic" pain and the pain-prone patient. *American Journal of Medicine,* 1959, **26,** 899–918.
24. Fabrega, H., Jr., and Manning, P. K. An integrated theory of disease: Ladino-Mestizo views of disease in the Chiapas Highlands. *Psychosomatic Medicine,* 1973, **35,** 223–239.
25. Fordyce, W. E., Fowler, R. S., Jr., Lehmann, J. F., and De Lateur, B. J. Some implications of learning in problems of chronic pain. *Journal of Chronic Diseases,* 1968, **21,** 179–190.
26. Fordyce, W. E., Fowler, R. S., Jr., Lehmann, J. F., De Lateur, B. J., Sand, P. L., and Trieschmann, R. B. Operant conditioning in the treatment of chronic pain. *Archives of Physical Medicine and Rehabilitation,* 1973, **54,** 399–408.
27. Friedman, A. S., Cowitz, B., Cohen, H. W., and Granick, S. Syndromes and themes of psychotic depression. *Archives of General Psychiatry,* 1963, **9,** 504–509.
28. Gannon, L., and Sternbach, R. A. Alpha enhancement as a treatment for pain: A case study. *Journal of Behavior Therapy and Experimental Psychiatry,* 1971, **2,** 209–213.
29. Graham, D. T. Health, disease, and the mind-body problem: Linguistic parallelism. *Psychosomatic Medicine,* 1967, **29,** 52–71.
30. Greenhoot, J. H. and Sternbach, R. A. Conjoint treatment of chronic pain. In J. J. Bonica (Ed.), *Advances in Neurology,* Vol. 4, *Pain.* New York: Raven Press, 1974.
31. Hamilton, M. A rating scale for depression. *Journal of Neurology and Psychiatry,* 1960, **23,** 56–62.
32. Harris, R. E., and Lingoes, J. C. Subscales for the Minnesota Multiphasic Personality Inventory: An aid to profile interpretation. Mimeographed materials. Department of Psychiatry, University of California, 1955.
33. Higgins, J. D., Tursky, B., and Schwartz, G. E. Shock-elicited pain and its reduction by concurrent tactile stimulation. *Science,* 1971, **172,** 866-867.
34. Jarvik, M. E. Drugs used in the treatment of psychiatric disorders. In L. S. Goodman and A. Gilman (Eds.), *The Pharmacological Basis of Therapeutics* (4th ed). New York: Macmillan, 1970.

35. Kay, D. W. K., Garside, R. F., Beamish, P., and Roy, J. R. Endogenous and neurotic syndromes of depression: A factor analytic study of 104 cases. Clinical features. *British Journal of Psychiatry*, 1969, **115**, 377–388.
36. Kear-Colwell, J. J. A taxonomy of depressive phenomena and its relationship to the reactive-endogenous dichotomy. *British Journal of Psychiatry*, 1972, **121**, 665–671.
37. Kenyon, F. E. Hypochondriasis: A clinical study. *British Journal of Psychiatry*, 1964, **110**, 478–488.
38. Kiloh, J. G., and Garside, R. F. The independence of neurotic depression and endogenous depression. *British Journal of Psychiatry*, 1963, **109**, 451–463.
39. Kreitman, N., Saisbury, P., Pearce, K., and Costain, W. R. Hypochondriasis and depression in out-patients at a general hospital. *British Journal of Psychiatry*, 1965, **111**, 607–615.
40. Ladee, G. A. *Hypochondriacal Syndromes.* Amsterdam: Elsevier, 1966.
41. Le Shan, L. The world of the patient in severe pain of long duration. *Journal of Chronic Diseases*, 1964, **17**, 119–126.
42. Lesse, S. The multivariant masks of depression. *American Journal of Psychiatry*, 1968, **124**, 35–40.
43. Liebeskind, J. C., Mayer, D. J., and Akil, H. Central mechanisms of pain inhibition: Studies of analgesia from focal brain stimulation. In J. J. Bonica (Ed.), *Advances in Neurology*, Vol. 4, *Pain.* New York: Raven Press, 1974.
44. Mayer, D. J., Wolfle, T. L., Akil, H., Carder, B., and Liebeskind, J. C. Analgesia from electrical stimulation in the brainstem of the rat. *Science*, 1971, **174**, 1351–1354.
45. Mechanic, D. The concept of illness behavior. *Journal of Chronic Diseases*, 1962, **15**, 189–194.
46. Mechanic, D. Social psychologic factors affecting the presentation of bodily complaints. *New England Journal of Medicine*, 1972, **286**, 1132–1139.
47. Melzack, R., and Schecter, B. Itch and vibration. *Science*, 1965, **147**, 1047–1048.
48. Melzack, R., and Wall, P. D. Pain mechanisms: A new theory. *Science*, 1965, **150**, 971–979.
49. Merskey, H. The characteristics of persistent pain in psychological illness. *Journal of Psychosomatic Research*, 1965, **9**, 291–298.
50. Merskey, H. Psychiatric patients with persistent pain. *Journal of Psychosomatic Research*, 1965, **9**, 299–309.
51. Merskey, H. Personality traits of psychiatric patients with pain. *Journal of Psychosomatic Research*, 1972, **16**, 163–166.
52. Merskey, H., and Hester, R. N. The treatment of chronic pain with psychotropic drugs. *Postgraduate Medical Journal*, 1972, **48**, 594–598.
53. Merskey, H., and Spear, F. G. *Pain: Psychological and Psychiatric Aspects.* London: Bailliere, Tindall & Cassell, 1967.
54. Overall, J. E. Dimensions of manifest depression. *Journal of Psychiatric Research*, 1962, **1**, 239-245.
55. Parbrook, G. D., Steel, D. F., and Dalrymple, D. G. Factors predisposing to postoperative pain and pulmonary complications. *British Journal of Anaesthesia*, 1973, **45**, 21–33.
56. Penman, J. Pain as an old friend. *Lancet*, 1954, **1**, 633–636.
57. Pilling, L. F., Brannick, T. L., and Swenson, W. M. Psychologic characteristics of psychiatric patients having pain as a presenting symptom. *Canadian Medical Association Journal*, 1967, **97**, 387–394.

58. Pilowsky, I. Dimensions of hypochondriasis. *British Journal of Psychiatry,* 1967, **113,** 89–93.
59. Pilowsky, I. The response to treatment in hypochondriacal disorders. *Australian and New Zealand Journal of Psychiatry,* 1968, **2,** 88–94.
60. Pilowsky, I. Abnormal illness behavior. *British Journal of Medical Psychology,* 1969, **42,** 347–351.
61. Pilowsky, I. The diagnosis of abnormal illness behavior. *Australian and New Zealand Journal of Psychiatry,* 1971, **5,** 136–138.
62. Pilowsky, I., and Bond, M. R. Pain and its management in malignant disease: Elucidation of staff-patient transactions. *Psychosomatic Medicine,* 1969, **31,** 400–404.
63. Pilowsky, I., Levine, S., and Boulton, D. M. The classification of depression by numerical taxonomy. *British Journal of Psychiatry,* 1969, **115,** 937–945.
64. Potter, S. *Three-upmanship: The Theory and Practice of Gamesmanship; Some Notes on Lifemanship; One upmanship.* New York: Holt, 1962.
65. Satran, R., and Goldstein, M. N. Pain perception: Modification of threshold of intolerance and cortical potentials by cutaneous stimulation. *Science,* 1973, **180,** 1201–1202.
66. Smith, G. M., and Beecher, H. K. Experimental production of pain in man. Sensitivity of a new method to 600 mg of aspirin. *Clinical Pharmacology and Therapeutics,* 1969, **10,** 213–216.
67. Smith, G. M., Egbert, L. D., Markowitz, R. A., Mosteller, F., and Beecher, H. K. An experimental pain method sensitive to morphine in man: The submaximum effort tourniquet technique. *Journal of Pharmacology and Experimental Therapeutics,* 1966, **154,** 324–332.
68. Smith, G. M., Lowenstein, E., Hubbard, J. H., and Beecher, H. K. Experimental pain produced by the submaximum effort tourniquet technique: Further evidence of validity. *Journal of Pharmacology and Experimental Therapeutics,* 1968, **163,** 468–474.
69. Stengel, E. Pain and the psychiatrist: The thirty-ninth Maudsley lecture. *British Journal of Psychiatry,* 1965, **111,** 795–802.
70. Sternbach, R. A. *Pain: A Psychophysiological Analysis.* New York: Academic Press, 1968.
71. Sternbach, R. A. Strategies and tactics in the treatment of patients with pain. In B. L. Crue, Jr. (Ed.), *Pain and Suffering: Selected Aspects.* Springfield, Ill.: Charles C. Thomas, 1970.
72. Sternbach, R. A. Varieties of pain games. In J. J. Bonica (Ed.), *Advances in Neurology,* Vol. 4, *Pain.* New York: Raven Press, 1974.
73. Sternbach, R. A. Pain and depression. In A. Kiev (Ed.), *Somatic Manifestations of Depressive Disorders,* Excerpta Medica, to be published.
74. Sternbach, R. A., Murphy, R. W., Akeson, W. H., and Wolf, S. R. Chronic low-back pain: The "low-back loser." *Postgraduate Medicine,* 1973, **53,** 135–138.
75. Sternbach, R. A., Murphy, R. W., Timmermans, G., Greenhoot, J. H., and Akeson, W. H. Measuring the severity of clinical pain. In J. J. Bonica (Ed.), *Advances in Neurology,* Vol. 4, *Pain.* New York: Raven Press, 1974.
76. Sternbach, R. A. and Rusk, T. N. Alternatives to the pain career. *Psychotherapy: Theory, Research and Practice,* 1973, **10,** 321–324.
77. Sternbach, R. A. and Tursky, B. On the psychophysical power function in electric shock. *Psychonomic Science,* 1964, **1,** 217–218.
78. Sternbach, R. A., and Tursky, B. Ethnic differences among housewives in psycho-

physical and skin potential responses to electric shock. *Psychophysiology*, 1965, **1**, 241–246.

79. Sternbach, R. A., Wolf, S. R., Murphy, R. W., and Akeson, W. H. Aspects of chronic low back pain. *Psychosomatics*, 1973, **14**, 52–56.
80. Sternbach, R. A., Wolf, S. R., Murphy, R. W., and Akeson, W. H. Traits of pain patients: The low-back "loser." *Psychosomatics*, 1973, **14**, 226–229.
81. Sullivan, R. Effect of different frequencies of vibration on pain-threshold detection. *Experimental Neurology*, 1968, **20**, 135–142.
82. Szasz, T. S. *Pain and Pleasure: A Study of Bodily Feelings.* New York: Basic Books, 1957.
83. Szasz, T. S. Language and pain. In S. Arieti (Ed.), *American Handbook of Psychiatry*, Vol. I. New York: Basic Books, 1959.
84. Szasz, T. S. The psychology of persistent pain: A portrait of l'homme douloureux. In A. Soulairac, J. Cahn, and J. Charpentier (Eds.), *Pain.* New York: Academic Press, 1968.
85. Taub, A., and Collins, W. F., Jr. Observation on the treatment of denervation dysesthesia with psychotropic agents. Postherpetic neuralgia, anesthesia dolorosa, peripheral neuropathy. In J. J. Bonica (Ed.), *Advances in Neurology*, Vol. 4, *Pain.* New York: Raven Press, 1974.
86. Tinling, D. C., and Klein, R. F. Psychogenic pain and aggression: The syndrome of the solitary hunter. *Psychosomatic Medicine*, 1966, **28**, 738–748.
87. Tursky, B., and Sternbach, R. A. Further physiological correlates of ethnic differences in responses to shock. *Psychophysiology*, 1967, **4**, 67–74.
88. Wall, P. D., and Sweet, W. H. Temporary abolition of pain in man. *Science*, 1967, **155**, 108–109.
89. Walters, A. Psychogenic regional pain alias hysterical pain. *Brain*, 1961, **84**(1), 1–18.
90. Watts, C. A. H. The mild endogenous depression. *British Medical Journal*, 1957, **1**, 4–8.
91. Wolff, B. B. Factor analysis of human pain responses: Pain endurance as a specific pain factor. *Journal of Abnormal Psychology*, 1971, **78**, 292–298.
92. Wolff, B. B. and Langley, S. Cultural factors and the response to pain: A review. *American Anthropologist*, 1968, **70**, 494–501.
93. Woodforde, J. M., and Merskey, H. Personality traits of patients with chronic pain. *Journal of Psychosomatic Research*, 1972, **16**, 167–172.
94. Woodforde, J. M., and Merskey, H. Some relationships between subjective measures of pain. *Journal of Psychosomatic Research*, 1972, **16**, 173–178.
95. Zborowski, M. *People in Pain.* San Francisco: Jossey–Bass, 1969.
96. Zung, W. W. K. A self-rating depression scale. *Archives of General Psychiatry*, 1965, **12**, 63–70.

Index